KU-393-523

Therapeutic Modalities for Sports Injuries

American Orthopaedic Society for Sports Medicine
Education Committee

Editor and Moderator:

David Drez, Jr., M.D.
Clinical Professor of Orthopedics
Louisiana State University Medical Center
New Orleans, Louisiana

GRIMSBY COLLEGE LIBRARY WITHDRAWN ... CORNER, GRIMSBY

Mosby Year Book

St. Louis Baltimore Boston Chicago London
Philadelphia Sydney Toronto

A Year Book Medical Publishers imprint of Mosby-
Year Book, Inc.

Mosby-Year Book, Inc., 11830 Westline Industrial
Drive, St. Louis, MO 63146.

Copyright © 1989 by Year Book Medical Publishers, Inc.
All rights reserved. No part of this publication may be
reproduced, stored in a retrieval system, or transmitted,
in any form or by any means—electronic, mechanical,
photocopying, recording, or otherwise—without prior
written permission from the publisher. Printed in the United
States of America.

2 3 4 5 6 7 8 9 0 R P 93 92 91

Library of Congress Cataloging-in-Publication Data

Therapeutic modalities for sports injuries / [edited by]
David Drez, Jr.
    p. cm.
  Based on a seminar sponsored by the Education
Committee of the American Orthopaedic Society for
Sports Medicine, held Dec. 12–14, 1986. Westin
O'Hare Hotel, Chicago, Ill.
  Bibliography: p.
  Includes index.
  ISBN 0-8151-2971-8
  1. Sports—Accidents and injuries—Treatment—
  Congresses.
I. Drez, David. II. American Orthopaedic Society for
Sports Medicine. Education Committee.
  [DNLM: 1. Athletic Injuries—therapy—
congresses.   QT 260 T3975 1986]
RD97.T48   1990
617.1'027—dc20   89-9052
DNLM/DLC   CIP
for Library of Congress

HE7
617·1027
ACC.
NO. A932244
02-6463

Sponsoring Editor: James D. Ryan
Assistant Director, Manuscript Services: Frances M.
 Perveiler
Proofroom Supervisor: Barbara M. Kelly

Contributors

Fred L. Allman, M.D.
Director of Sports Medicine
Medical Center Orthopaedic
   Resident Training
   Program
Atlanta, Georgia

Jack T. Andrish, M.D.
Staff Surgeon
Department of Orthopedic
   Surgery
Cleveland Clinic Foundation
Cleveland, Ohio

Jay S. Cox, M.D.
Associate Professor of
   Surgery
Uniformed Services
   University for the Health
   Sciences
Orthopaedic Consultant
U.S. Naval Academy
Annapolis, Maryland

Walton W. Curl, M.D.
Assistant Professor of
   Orthopedics
Bowman Gray School of
   Medicine
Wake Forest University
Winston-Salem, North
   Carolina

Robert D. D'Ambrosia, M.D.
Professor and Chairman
Department of Orthopaedics
Louisiana State University
   School of Medicine
New Orleans, Louisiana

Dale M. Daniel, M.D.
Associate Clinical Professor
   of Orthopedics
University of California at
   San Diego
San Diego, California

Jesse C. DeLee,
   B.S., M.D.
Clinical Associate Professor
The University of Texas
   Health Science Center at
   San Antonio
San Antonio, Texas

Ben Graf, M.D.
Assistant Professor
Division of Orthopaedic
   Surgery
University of Wisconsin
Madison, Wisconsin

William A. Grana, M.D.
*Director, Oklahoma Center
for Athletes
Clinical Professor of
Orthopedic Surgery and
Rehabilitation
University of Oklahoma
College of Medicine
Oklahoma City, Oklahoma*

George F.
Hewson, Jr., M.D.
*Clinic Lecturer
Team Physician and
Orthopaedic Consultant
University of Arizona
St. Mary's Hospital
Tucson, Arizona*

James G. Howe, M.D.
*Associate Professor
University of Vermont
Chief of Service
Medical Center Hospital of
Vermont
Burlington, Vermont*

Robert E. Hunter, M.D.
*Associate Professor
Department of Orthopedic
Surgery
Director, University of
Minnesota Sports
Medicine Institute
University of Minnesota
Hospital and Clinics
Minneapolis, Minnesota*

Peter A. Indelicato, M.D.
*Associate Professor and
Chief of Sports Medicine
University of Florida
Gainesville, Florida*

Lyle J. Micheli, M.D.
*Assistant Clinical Professor
of Orthopaedic Surgery
Harvard Medical School
Director, Division of Sports
Medicine
Children's Hospital
Boston, Massachusetts*

Lonnie Paulos, M.D.
*University of Utah Hospital
L.D.S. Hospital
Salt Lake City, Utah*

Bruce Reider, M.D.
*Associate Professor of
Surgery
University of Chicago
Director of Sports Medicine
University of Chicago
Chicago, Illinois*

Kenneth Singer, M.D.
*Clinical Senior Instructor of
Surgery
Division of Orthopedic
Surgery and
Rehabilitation
University of Oregon Health
Sciences Center
Staff Orthopedic Surgeon
Sacred Heart General
Hospital
Eugene, Oregon*

William D. Stanish, M.D.,
F.R.C.S.(C.), F.A.C.S.
*Associate Professor of
Surgery
Dalhousie University
Orthopaedic Surgeon
Victoria General Hospital
Halifax, Nova Scotia*

J. Richard Steadman, M.D.
*American Academy of
  Orthopaedic Surgeons
American College of Sports
  Medicine
Staff Surgeon
Barton Memorial Hospital
South Lake Tahoe, California*

W. Michael Walsh, M.D.
*Associate Professor
Director of Sports Medicine
Department of Orthopaedic
  Surgery and
  Rehabilitation
University of Nebraska
  Medical Center
Omaha, Nebraska*

Edward M. Wojtys, M.D.
*Assistant Professor
Department of Orthopaedic
  Surgery
University of Michigan
  Medical School
Ann Arbor, Michigan*

G. William Woods, M.D.
*Clinical Associate Professor
  of Orthopedic Surgery
Baylor College of Medicine
The Methodist Hospital
Houston, Texas*

Preface

The Education Committee of the American Orthopaedic Society for Sports Medicine was concerned about the lack of objective data on the modalities that have been used in both the treatment and rehabilitation of musculoskeletal injuries. A proposal was made to the Board of Directors of the American Orthopaedic Society for Sports Medicine regarding sponsorship of a seminar to evaluate objectively the data that were available on these modalities.

The objectives of the seminar were to (1) identify and classify the modalities, (2) define the mechanism of action of each modality, (3) give the indications and contraindications for use of modalities, (4) provide scientific documentation regarding the use of modalities, and (5) identify areas of needed research.

A general classification of modalities and a general outline of the program was done by the seminar chairman. Moderators were selected for the evaluation teams, and their role was to amplify and further define presentations that were needed in each area. The evaluation teams gathered information on the specific modalities and prepared the information that they were able to obtain for presentation to the entire seminar group. Time was allotted for colloquium that would be an open discussion for formulation of conclusions. Evaluation teams were then to meet and prepare a report in the areas in which they were assigned. Following this, the completed reports were prepared for publication.

The report that follows represents the collected endeavors of those who gave of their time to bring this project to completion. Many hours were spent by the participants in researching and referencing this material.

Any conclusions or recommendations from this seminar report are not to be interpreted as standards, guidelines, or endorsements by the American Orthopaedic Society for Sports Medicine. This seminar was held solely for the purpose of educating, reporting of timely information, and stimulating research in this area.

Special thanks are due to Carol Rosegay and to Sanford J. Hill of the American Orthopaedic Society for Sports Medicine for their help, to Marti Daigle for her tireless efforts in the preparation of the typescript, and to program participants for giving their time.

David Drez, Jr., M.D.

Contents

1

Heat Modalities

Jay S. Cox, M.D.

Jack T. Andrish, M.D.

Peter A. Indelicato, M.D.

W. Michael Walsh, M.D.

INTRODUCTION

Treatment by heat modalities, i.e., "thermotherapy," is therapy that attempts to increase the temperature of tissue. The transmission of heat to tissue occurs by three mechanisms: conduction, convection, and radiation. Conduction involves the exchange of thermal energy between two surfaces in physical contact with each other (example, hot packs). Convection, a more rapid process than conduction, occurs when air or water molecules move across the body, creating temperature variations (example, whirlpool). Radiation is the transfer of heat from a warm source to a cooler source through a conducting medium such as air. The physiological effects of heat are discussed below.

Analgesic Effect.—This mechanism is not fully understood, but it is known that heat acts selectively on free nerve endings, tissues, and peripheral nerve fibers, increasing the pain threshold. Ultrasound at intermediate levels will decrease sensory nerve conduction velocity. Heat will relieve muscle spasm by directly effecting gamma fibers of muscle spindles, thereby decreasing the spindle activity and sensitivity to stretch. Heat applied to the body surface may produce a decrease in the spasm due to reflex action through the thermal receptors. Also, it has been postulated that heat can activate descending pain inhibitory systems. (The vasodilatation that occurs from application of heat reduces pain by removing the byproducts of injured tissue, which include prostaglandin, histamine, and bradykinin. These metabolites stimulate the nerve fibers that cause the pain-spasm-pain cycle.)

Vascular Changes.—Heat causes vasodilatation, which also results in the analgesia. Heat also increases nutrition at the cellular level and removes metabolites of the inflammatory process.

Metabolism.—The metabolism of tissues is dependent upon temperature. As blood flow increases to tissues due to a rise in temperature, so does the supply of oxygen, and, therefore, the metabolic rate. Increased blood flow also brings a larger number of antibodies, leukocytes, nutrients, and enzymes to tissue. For each 10°C rise in temperature, the cells' chemical activity and the metabolic rate will increase two to three times.

Increase in Extensibility of Collagen Tissue.—Heat alters the viscoelastic properties of collagen tissue. There is residual elongation of the tissue. However, this elongation can be of therapeutic benefit only if it can be maintained when used in conjunction with strength. Joint stiffness is also relieved.

Summary

The physiological effects of heat are *increased*...

- Local temperature (superficially and deep depending on the modality)

- Local metabolism

- Vasodilatation of arterioles and capillaries

- Blood flow to the part heated

- Leukocytes and phagocytosis

- Capillary permeability

- Axon reflex activity

- Lymphatic and venous drainage

- Removal of metabolic wastes

- Elasticity of ligaments, capsular fibers, and muscles

- Analgesia

- Formation of edema

and *decreased*...

- Muscle tone

- Muscle spasm.

The discussions that follow will evaluate the superficial heat modalities, diathermy, and ultrasound in detail.

CLASSIFICATION, MECHANISM, AND ACTION OF SUPERFICIAL HEAT MODALITIES

Superficial heat modalities are those physical modalities that provide an increase in heat, which produces a subsequent increase in circulation to a depth no greater than 1 cm. These include warm whirlpool, contrast baths, paraffin baths, hydrocollator packs, and infrared heat. Each modality will be discussed briefly under the clinical application subheading.

Studies show that application of superficial heat to the skin, irrespective of form, will cause a rather sudden rise in the superficial skin temperature. Heat will also increase the blood flow in a specific area secondary to the increase in temperature, which in turn may increase the supply of oxygen, antibodies, and white cells to an area of damaged soft tissue. The clearing of harmful metabolites is also facilitated with this increased blood flow.

In addition to the advantage of providing more nutrients to an area of damaged tissue, superficial heat appears to provide a beneficial analgesic effect. The exact mechanism of this analgesia is unknown, but perhaps the equalization of the temperature gradient between the injured and uninjured tissues is a factor.

Indications

The indications for the use of superficial heat are those conditions that benefit from an increase in circulation, the relaxation of muscle spasm, and an increase in extensibility of joint stiffness. Due to the possibility of increasing extracellular edema, one should not apply heat to a recently injured area for up to 48 to 72 hours following the trauma. The general indications for superficial heat application are to...

- Reduce pain and stiffness

- Alleviate muscle spasm

- Increase range of motion of a joint

- Accelerate metabolic processes

- Resolve hematoma

- Relieve contracture.

Contraindications

Patients with...

- Impaired sensation for pain or temperature in local or regional areas

- Impaired skin circulation or scar

- Malignancy

- Acute inflammation, trauma, or neurologic impairment

- Poor thermal regulation.

CAUTION: Heat is contraindicated for semicomatose or elderly patients or infants who cannot report reactions.

Clinical Application

Warm Whirlpools.—Position the patient as comfortably as possible in the whirlpool. The directions of flow must be within 6 to 8 in. of the area of the body that is to be treated. In general, the temperature of the water should be between 36 and 43°C. For a single extremity, the water temperature should be between 36 and 40°C and between 36 and 41°C for the full body. Usually 15 to 20 minutes immersion in warm water is considered optimal. If patients can perform mild exercise while the treated extremity or body is immersed, they can increase the blood flow to the deeper structures. When increased blood flow to a muscle is considered the end goal, modest exercise will best accomplish this rather than the application of superficial heat.

Contrast Baths.—The patient's injured area is immersed in water, alternating between warm and cold water tanks. The warm water temperature should be between 40.5 and 43.3°C. The recommended cold water temperature is between 10°C and 15.5°C. The involved area should be immersed in the warm water tank for approximately five minutes and then in the cold water tank for approximately one to two minutes. The process should continue for a total of 30 minutes. In order to minimize the possibility of swelling, the final cycle of alternating hot and cold should end in the cold water tank. This form of contrast heating and cooling allegedly stimulates circulation and produces a hyperemia by alternating vasodilatation and vasoconstriction of the superficial blood vessels. Theoretically, the process produces a maximum increase of blood flow to the involved area.

Paraffin Wax.—Paraffin baths are a simple and somewhat efficient, albeit messy, technique in applying a fairly high degree of localized heat to the smaller joints of our body, particularly the wrist, hand, ankle, and foot. Paraffin wax provides approximately six times more heat than normal water (because the added mineral oil in the paraffin lowers the melting point of the paraffin). Most baths contain 7 parts wax to 1 part mineral oil at 52 to 54°C. The method of application of paraffin wax is divided into two general categories—dipping and wrapping. Dipping involves immersing the extremity into the paraffin for a few seconds and then removing it to allow the paraffin to harden. This procedure is repeated until several layers have been accumulated on the involved area. Wrapping consists of dipping the involved area in the paraffin until it becomes coated and then wrapping the involved area in a plastic bag with several layers of towels to act as an insulator. The treatment should continue for at least 20 to 30 minutes. Risk of burns in paraffin baths is substantially higher than with other forms of superficial heat.

Hydrocollator Packs.—These commercially available canvas pouches of petroleum distillate are a common form of superficial heat in clinics. The thermostat maintains a temperature of between 50 and 70°C. Commercially produced padding towels for the packs provide approximately 2.5 cm of padding (which is recommended to prevent superficial burns). Treatment with hydrocollator packs should last between 15 and 20 minutes.

Infrared Heat.—Effectiveness from this form of heat application and moist hot packs seems to be essentially the same. However, infrared heat only penetrates a few millimeters of the skin. Two of the advantages of an infrared lamp are that superficial temperatures rise quite rapidly and the unit does not come in contact with the patient. Superficial skin burns can occur because of the intense infrared radiation. To avoid these burns, a warm moist towel should be applied over the body segment being treated. In addition, protective toweling should be placed around the areas that are not being treated. The patient should be positioned approximately 20 inches from the source. Treatment should last approximately 15 to 20 minutes. The skin should be checked every few minutes to prevent superficial burning.

Conclusion

As a result of superficial heat application, various physiological changes occur that result in increased circulation and reduction of pain and muscle spasm. Although the development of these heat modalities is based, in part, on basic science information and the understanding of the physiological response to heat application, there remains a great need to investigate further the exact mechanisms of action and the effectiveness of each of the superficial heat modalities.

LIBRARY

CLINICAL EFFECTS OF DIATHERMY: SHORTWAVE AND MICROWAVE

Diathermy (the use of high frequency electromagnetic currents) induces deep heating in biologic tissues by vibration and distortion of the tissue molecules.

Classification

Shortwave diathermy came into clinical use in the 1920s. The purpose of shortwave diathermy is to induce local hyperemia in tissues and to produce analgesia and decrease muscle spasms by sedation of sensory and motor nerves. These effects are mediated through induction of deep heat within the tissues. Well-designed experimental studies in the literature outline the depth of penetration of heat generated by diathermy. Heating of tissues occurs to a depth of 3 to 5 cm. However, the majority of the heat is dissipated superficially within the subcutaneous fat. Indeed, probably a good portion of the heating of the superficial layer of muscle is conducted from the adjacent heated subcutaneous fat. A principle of diathermy relates that water-rich tissues, such as muscle and fat, serve as good conductors and are heated preferentially.

Shortwave diathermy can be applied through a capacitive field or an induction field method. In the capacitive arrangement, the patient is placed between two plate electrodes to complete a circuit. The inductive arrangement uses the magnetic field of a coil to couple the patient into the shortwave diathermy circuit.

Indications

Whenever deep heating of subcutaneous tissue and superficial muscle layers is desired, for example:

- Osteoarthritis

- Rheumatoid arthritis

- Bursitis

- Tendonitis

- Strains

- Sprains

- Neuritis.

Contraindications

Patients with:

- Fresh hemorrhage in tissues

- Sensory loss (One complication of diathermy is overheating and tissue burns. A patient with inadequate sensation, then, cannot tell if a burn is being produced acutely.)

- Moist dressings (Moisture, including perspiration, can concentrate the effects from diathermy and lead to local burns.)

- Ischemia (Since diathermy induces heat and at the same time increases local tissue metabolism, ischemia can lead to further tissue damage by increasing the metabolic demands on preexisting metabolically marginal tissues.)

- Arteriosclerosis

- Phlebitis

- Metallic implants (Metal can concentrate the heat effects from diathermy, producing overheating of metal and injury to the surrounding local tissues.)

- Cardiac pacemakers (Because of the electromagnetic radiation, electronic or magnetic equipment can malfunction when exposed to diathermy. Other electronic devices such as hearing aids and watches should be removed.)

• Epiphyseal plates in children

• Any metal in contact with skin

• Tumor

• Intrauterine devices

• Gonads

• Pelvic area in menstruating females (Diathermy may produce menorrhagia.)

• Pregnancy

• Infection

• Contact eye lenses.

Complications

Burns can result from overheating. Most commonly this occurs as subcutaneous fat necrosis, which can result from patient movement during treatments, improper technique (improper set up of the induction coils), faulty equipment, or inadequate supervision.

Microwave Diathermy

Microwave diathermy refers to high frequency electromagnetic radiation used to induce deep heat within biologic tissues. In general, microwaves do not penetrate tissue as deeply as shortwave and ultrasound. The indications, contraindications, and clinical applications of microwave diathermy are identical to shortwave diathermy.

General Principles of Application for Diathermy

The patient should lie on a wooden table or sit in a wooden chair. No metal should touch the patient during the diathermy applications. The duration of each individual treatment will average 20 minutes. For acute problems the frequency of treatments may be once or twice a day for 10 to 14 days. Chronic problems will require treatments three times a week for 10 to 14 days. If a second series of treatments is indicated, a minimum 2-week interval between the series is recommended.

Safety

Numerous scientific studies on the effects of electromagnetic radiation from shortwave and microwave diathermy units have demonstrated that these methods of heat application are safe. Therapists can receive doses of electromagnetic radiation above the recommended maximum limits ($10 \mu W/sq cm \times 8$ hours/day), but they would be extremely negligent for such excessive exposure to happen.

Clinical Effectiveness

Farrell and Twomey (1982) carried out a controlled clinical trial investigating microwave diathermy plus abdominal strengthening exercises and activity modification (ergonomics) vs. a regimen of passive spinal mobilization and manipulation. Forty-eight patients were included in this study. The results demonstrated that those patients with manipulations took significantly less time until they were symptom-free ($P < .001$). However, 91% of *all* subjects had recovered in 4 weeks.

The *Journal of the American Medical Association* (1983) under their Diagnostic and Therapeutic Technology Assessment stated: "There have been no convincing trials comparing one type of diathermy with the other or ... with hot packs."

Perhaps the best controlled study on clinical effectiveness of diathermy was by Gibson et al. (1985). This was a controlled comparison of shortwave diathermy treatment with osteopathic treatment in patients with nonspecific low back pain. Shortwave diathermy was compared with a placebo diathermy as well as to the spinal (osteopathic) manipulation treatment group. One hundred nine patients were included in this study and randomly assigned into one of these three treatment protocols. The average age was 34 to 40 years. Tumors, spondylolysis, spondylolisthesis, inflammatory disease, and metabolic disease were excluded as etiologies for the low back pain. Results of this study demonstrated that greater than 50% of subjects in each group received benefits from treatments. Significant improvements were noted in all groups at the end of the 2-week treatment period. Further, these improvements were maintained at the time of patient review at 12 weeks. The physicians who evaluated the patients at the end of 12 weeks were "blinded" to the treatment category of the patient. The results were unrelated to the initial severity of pain. A significant reduction in the number of patients requiring analgesic medication was found only in the placebo group. Indeed, important in this study was the fact that neither manipulation nor shortwave diathermy was superior to placebo alone. The authors emphasize that regular contact between the patient and the therapist is probably the greatest benefit—the patients' conditions improved quicker than the natural history would otherwise suggest. This article also quotes several other multicenter trials in the literature that have compared the manipulations with various physical therapy modalities and have shown no significant difference or advantage of one over the other.

Clinical Conclusions for Shortwave/Microwave Diathermy

• Diathermy can provide heating of biologic tissues.

- Tissues heated can be 3-cm to 5-cm deep.

- Fat can be selectively heated, which can at times lead to burn and fat necrosis.

- The *clinical* value of diathermy is probably through a *placebo effect*.

THERAPEUTIC ULTRASOUND

While the clinical use of ultrasound is a product of the 20th century, the principles upon which this modality are based go back to the middle of the 19th century. For example, Joule in 1847 discovered that high-frequency electricity could be used to produce high-frequency sound energy. In 1880, the Curies reported that certain asymmetrical crystals possessed electrical properties. They showed that deformation of these crystalline structures created a measurable current known as the piezoelectric effect. This phenomenon is well known to orthopedic surgeons because of its implication for electrical stimulation of bone healing. However, the corollary of that discovery was the so-called reverse piezoelectric effect, which states that if an electrical current is applied across the face of certain crystals, the crystal can be made to deform or ultimately resonate. Over a half-century ago the potentially destructive aspect of ultrasound energy was stumbled upon by Chilowsky and Langevin (1916) when they noted that fish swimming into the path of an ultrasonic beam were instantly killed. In 1927, Wood and Loomis were also able to demonstrate disruption of other types of living cells by ultrasound energy. In 1937 the first report on tissue effects by ultrasound was published. This study suggested that there were both beneficial as well as harmful effects to be seen. This resulted in the first reported use of ultrasound as a therapeutic modality in 1938, when a case report was published describing the use of ultrasound to treat sciatica. After being temporarily sidetracked by World War II, interest in ultrasound for medical purposes burgeoned in the late 1940s and 1950s. In the 1950s we can truly say that the medical use of therapeutic ultrasound came into wide acceptance.

As its name implies, ultrasound is any high-frequency sound that is above the range heard by the human ear. In general, ultrasound is considered to be any sound with a frequency of 20,000 cycles per second (20,000 Hz) or higher. Ultrasound in comparison with other heat modalities is unique in that it is part of the acoustic spectrum and not the electromagnetic spectrum. Every other member of the group of heating modalities uses electromagnetic energy to produce the heating effect. Consequently, all heating modalities share certain common characteristics, but ultrasound has many different characteristics. For example, electromagnetic energy is transmitted best in a vacuum, while ultrasound is not transmitted at all in a vacuum. Electromagnetic energy travels theoretically at the speed of light, 300 *million* meters per second, while the average velocity of ultrasound at sea level pressure is 330 meters per second. Ultrasonic energy is almost entirely absorbed by the major components of our atmosphere (nitrogen, oxygen, and carbon dioxide); hence, the need for some type of coupling medium between the ultrasonic generator and the human body. If the ultrasonic applicator were placed directly on the skin, even the small amounts of air trapped in the pores of the skin would absorb the ultrasound and make its use unpredictable and unfeasible.

As a heat modality, ultrasound displays several important characteristics. A property important to clinical use of ultrasound is that the penetration of human tissues by ultrasonic energy is inversely proportional to the frequency of the ultrasound generated. Another extremely important characteristic is that the more homogeneous the material, the more readily the ultrasonic energy penetrates the material, such as subcutaneous fat. Fat acts as a tremendous insulator for all of the electromagnetic forms of energy. Consequently, none of the other heating modalities penetrate deep within the body, but because ultrasound is attenuated to only a small degree by subcutaneous fat, it reaches the deeper tissues. Another characteristic of ultrasound is that in comparison to the electromagnetic spectrum, ultrasound uses energy of shortwave length. Wavelength is directly related to velocity; ultrasound uses energy 1,000,000 times slower than electromagnetic energy. These much shorter wavelengths are important in producing the effects discussed in other parts of this presentation.

In simple terms, ultrasound energy is generated by the machines that we see every day in our hospitals and clinics by the following method. A 60-Hz, 110-V house current is run through an oscillating circuit that changes the back-and-forth flow of the electricity. Instead of 60 cycles per second, the electricity now alternates at a rate that will produce the maximum excursion for whatever crystal material it is attached to. This particular frequency for each material is known as the resonant frequency. This high-frequency electricity then continues through a step-up transformer to produce an intermediate voltage on modern ultrasound machines of some 200 to 300 V. This modified electromagnetic energy is coupled to the crystal, usually by a coaxial cable. While quartz crystals were originally used, the two common synthetic crystals in use today are barium titanate and lead zirconate. These crystals are bonded to a metal or glass facing, which is applied to the patient surface by way of an intervening coupling agent such as mineral oil, water, or the now available commercially manufactured gels. The most common ultrasound generators in clinical use today operate at a frequency of about 1 mHz. This frequency represents a compromise between the ability of ultrasonic energy to penetrate tissues (lower frequencies penetrate farther) and the ability to create thermal vs. nonthermal effects (high frequency gives greater thermal effect).

While a number of textbooks predicted we would experience much greater use of lower frequency (90 kHz) machines in the 1980s, these predictions apparently have not come true. Instead, we see more research being directed at the clinical use of higher frequency (3 mHz) generators because of their unique properties. At least one major manufacturer now makes a generator that can be switched back and forth from approximately 1 mHz to 3 mHz. The surface area of the ultrasound head (in square centimeters) is used to describe the *intensity* of ultrasound applied to the patient. This intensity (in W/sq cm) can be set roughly on the ultrasound machine. Usual clinical intensities vary from 0.5 W/sq cm to 2.0 W/sq cm. Actually, the sensation of warmth many times is used to determine optimal intensity; for example, a deep aching pain indicates overheating of periosteum. Pulsing the ultrasound (energy being applied during 20% to 50% of the cycle) also can be used to decrease overall intensity and the thermal effects.

Standard physical therapy textbooks, such as the second edition of Griffin and Karselis (1982), contain some indication of reliance on anecdotal evidence and "clinical experience" to substantiate some of the purported effects of ultrasound. More recently, some of these alleged effects have been studied by substantial research efforts. For example, the most recent textbook on the subject by Michlovitz, entitled *Thermal Agents in Rehabilitation* (1986), takes a much more critical look at some of the long-held beliefs in regard to ultrasound and points out that these effects may or may not be true. As a matter of convenience, we can categorize the effects of ultrasound as thermal, nonthermal, neural, connective tissue, and mineral deposit effects. Each one of these will be discussed briefly.

Thermal Effects.—As an ultrasound beam travels through any given tissue, the energy is either conducted, absorbed, or reflected. Absorption of ultrasound energy gives the thermal or heating effect. The ready conduction of ultrasound energy through subcutaneous fat can produce temperature increases in deep tissue. Since penetration is inversely proportional to frequency, 1-mHz ultrasound will easily heat tissues at a depth of 5 cm, while 90-kHz ultrasound will heat tissues at a depth of 10 cm. Furthermore, it is a fact that ultrasound can produce this tissue temperature rise in the shortest span of treatment time. Because of the dense homogeneous nature of metal, most of the ultrasound energy is conducted through the metallic implant and is not reflected. Therefore, no increased thermal effects are seen when ultrasound is used over metallic devices. Common figures given in the literature are that muscle temperature will rise 1 to 2°C in 20 to 30 seconds of ultrasound application. During that same time, bone temperature may increase 5 to 6°C. Approximately 35% of ultrasound energy is reflected from cortical bone. This reflected energy, as well as the energy absorbed at the bone periosteum interface, can result in significant overheating of the periosteum. However, this occurs in an irregular fashion, causing "hot spots" that may produce burning of the tissues. Another well-documented thermal effect of ultrasound is an increased local blood flow within the warmed tissues.

Nonthermal Effects.—This is probably the most popular area of ultrasound research at the moment. Clearly, ultrasound affects living tissue in ways that have nothing to do with tissue temperature rise. Ultrasound appears to alter diffusion of sodium and potassium ions and probably ionic calcium as well. Also, alterations appear to take place in cell permeability, perhaps accounting for some of these diffusion differences. Some of the other nonthermal effects derive from the radiation pressure changes that occur within the tissues. One of the best-documented and potentially harmful effects is cavitation—the phenomenon in which gas bubbles trapped within the tissues in the field of ultrasonic energy enlarge and vibrate in response to the ultrasonic waves. These vibrating bubbles set up motion in the cellular fluids surrounding them and create a fluid movement phenomenon known as acoustic microstreaming. Streaming that takes place away from the source of acoustic energy in response to radiation pressure changes is the basis for the use of phonophoresis. Another descriptive term used for many years (though much less in recent writings) to illustrate these acoustic pressure changes is the "micromassage effect."

Neural Effects.—An analgesic effect has long been ascribed to the use of ultrasound. This is one claim that seems largely anecdotal. Certainly the mechanism of any pain reduction is not clear at present. There may be some reduction of pain through the thermal effect of ultrasound. Some of the known effects of ultrasonic energy on nerve tissue may also be at least partially responsible for the analgesic phenomenon. The peripheral nerve contains more corticosteroid than any other human soft tissue except the adrenal cortex. Research has shown an increase in its corticosteroid content following ultrasonic irradiation. Effects of ultrasound on nerve conduction are not clearly established. According to Ter Haar and Dyson (1981): "In some cases, ultrasound can completely block the action potential, and in others it can increase the amplitude of the depolarization spike." Farmer (1968) reported a definite change in conduction velocity with ultrasound exposure. With intermediate intensities of ultrasound between 0.5 and 1.5 W/sq cm, conduction velocity decreases. At intensities below 0.5 or above 2 W/sq cm, conduction velocity increases. Whether this change has some direct role in the reduction of pain remains to be proven. Another fertile field for investigation seems to be the use of ultrasonic energy in the treatment of nerve injury.

Connective Tissue Effects.—Numerous *clinical* reports indicate that ultrasound is effective in diminishing the pain of neuromas and adhesive scars. Griffin and Karselis (1982) reported that where such pain is due to excess proliferation of connective tissue, relief of pain may be due to relaxation of polypeptide bonds after the absorption of ultrasonic energy.

The use of ultrasound to aid in tissue healing is another area of intense research interest. Much work has been done on this topic in England. Studies show the usefulness of ultrasound in promoting the healing of pressure sores and varicose ulcers. Treatment by ultrasound during the inflammatory phase of tissue repair appears to be particularly beneficial, probably through the effect of ultrasound on mast cells and macrophages. It seems clear that, through some mechanism, ultrasound will stimulate fibroblast activity in the synthesis of reparative tissue. It should be pointed out that much of the recent work on ultrasound-induced tissue healing is conducted with 3-mHz ultrasound, a frequency that has not been widely used in the United States up to this time. Ultrasound will increase the extensibility of tendon, as well as aiding in the stretching of joint contractures. These effects are probably thermal in nature. Ultrasound appears to be more practical and helpful than other forms of heat because of its deep penetrating quality.

Elevation of tissue temperature probably accounts for the ability of ultrasound to reduce muscle spasm. The exact mechanisms are not clear, but thermal effects may alter muscle contractility, reduce muscle spindle activity, or simply reduce pain, which breaks the pain-spasm-pain cycle.

Mineral Deposition Effects.—This is probably the most unsubstantiated of all claims regarding ultrasound treatments. While many statements have been made that ultrasound can increase the resorption of calcific deposits in soft tissue, as yet, no controlled studies using serial roentgenograms have supported this theory. More likely, the ultrasound in such cases relieves pain and other symptoms rather than objectively decreasing the presence of calcium in the tissues.

Phonophoresis

The radiation pressure changes that accompany ultrasound energy have the ability to drive intact large complex molecules through the skin and into the deeper tissues. Some researchers, according to Griffin and Kar-selis (1982), claim recovery of significant amounts of ultrasound-driven medications as deep as 10 cm within the tissues after 5 minutes of treatment. Such compounds as corticosteroids, salicylates, and local anesthetics can be delivered in this fashion. In fact, it appears that phonophoresis is one of the most helpful substantiated uses of ultrasound.

Indications for Ultrasound

The prime indication for the use of ultrasound is any condition in which deep and prompt tissue heating is needed. This would include the desire to produce thermal-related vasodilation. If the desired site of treatment is 2 cm or more beneath the skin's surface, ultrasound seems especially suitable as a heating modality. This primary indication for ultrasound makes it useful in a wide variety of both articular and extraarticular musculoskeletal pathologies. One caveat, though, is that no direct antiinflammatory effect of ultrasound alone has ever been demonstrated. Consequently, it is difficult to understand why pain would be reduced in inflammatory conditions such as bursitis.

Treatment of adhesions of hypotrophic scars, especially those limiting range of motion of joints, are amenable to treatment with ultrasound. Research has substantiated a role for ultrasound in the treatment of pressure sores. Substantial clinical evidence exists that ultrasound is highly effective in decreasing the pain of neuromas. Ultrasound has been used in the treatment of plantar warts. Also, use of ultrasound in treating a large organized hematoma continues to be listed as an indication in standard physical therapy texts. However, there is no basic science research that supports the ability of ultrasound to alter the hematoma.

Contraindications

The contraindication to use of ultrasound occurs when one does *not* want to produce a tissue temperature rise. Therefore, ultrasound is contraindicated...

- Immediately following trauma when bleeding is prominent.

- In the thoracic region when the patient has a cardiac pacemaker.

- Over areas of suspected malignancy.

- Over open growth plates in children.

- Over the eye, the heart, the pregnant uterus, or the testes.

Authors differ in their recommendations regarding the use of ultrasound over areas of suspected thrombophlebitis. The use should either be avoided altogether or at least kept to extremely low intensities. Ultrasound should be used with great caution over areas that have either decreased sensation or less than normal arterial circulation.

Clinical Applications

The standard moving head technique using mineral oil or commercially available gel at relatively moderate intensities (no greater than 1.5 W/sq cm) is the most common method for most clinical applications of ultrasound. The moving head helps reduce undesired overheating of tissue. The stationary technique of application is being used less and less, probably because of the inherent uneven transmission of ultrasound from the transducer. Pulsed ultrasound with a duty cycle of 20 to 50% is another standard technique of reducing undesired overheating. Underwater ultrasound has been used, especially in the treatment of pressure sores or over irregular bony areas. In this case, the transducer is held 0.5 to 3.0 cm from the body's surface, but accumulated air bubbles on the transducer face must be intermittently removed. Another method of application uses a balloon filled with water or gel, which is attached to the transducer itself. The balloon provides the coupling between the transducer and irregular bony surfaces. Phonophoresis is a standard application of ultrasound at this time. However, there are no controlled studies to date giving specific dose-related effects of the phonophoresis technique.

Summary

Ultrasound is a unique physical modality in that it uses high-frequency sound energy to produce both thermal and nonthermal effects in human tissues. Then, if we define the term "effective" as having a definite discernible impact on biologic tissues, then ultrasonic energy is definitely effective. It has a clear and prompt thermal effect at greater depth than any of the electromagnetic heating modalities. Whether all of the described beneficial results of such known effects really occur remains a point for some debate and further research. Of particular interest should be further investigation into the less well-defined nonthermal effects of ultrasonic energy.

HEAT MODALITIES: RECOMMENDATIONS FOR FURTHER RESEARCH

We recommend that scientific research be conducted to determine if the application of superficial heat can decrease the soft-tissue healing time. It appears that the actual healing time cannot be influenced by superficial heat, but this should be addressed scientifically. Research should be done to evaluate the resolution of the inflammatory process and...

- To determine if hydrocortisone or corticosteroids have any effect on the strength of a tendon. An animal model could be developed to study the tensile strength of either the patella tendon or the Achilles tendon. Hydrocortisone ointment with ultrasound, i.e., phonophoresis, is a popular modality in physical therapy. The application should be evaluated scientifically.

- To determine if skin discoloration as observed and sometimes associated with phonophoresis could be prevented. Studies should be conducted to examine the factors and methods of prevention.

- To determine dose and dosages of heat modalities in relation to their corresponding healing responses.

- To determine the optimum time to switch from cold therapy to heat therapy. It is commonly recommended that after 48 hours, heat therapy should be started, as opposed to cold modalities. To determine if this is true or not, a study should be conducted with an animal model, to examine the various applications of cold followed by heat in regard to edema, bleeding, and tissue response.

2 | Cold Modalities

William A. Grana, M.D.

Walton L. Curl, M.D.

Bruce Reider, M.D.

CRYOTHERAPY

Cryotherapy is the treatment of injury or disease with cold. This section does not include discussion of cryosurgery, the use of cold to ablate tissue; it focuses on the therapeutic effects of cold following musculo-skeletal injury.

The result of musculoskeletal injury is hemorrhage, inflammation, edema, muscle spasm, and pain. The physiological effects of injury produce the loss of motion, disuse, deconditioning, and, ultimately, loss of function.

Cold is a widely used physical agent, the use of which is based primarily on clinical and empirical evidence. It is used for the immediate care and rehabilitation of soft-tissue injuries as well as other kinds of musculoskeletal problems. In this discussion, *immediate care* is defined as the first 48 hours and *rehabilitation* is the period of time following the first 48 hours of injury. The use of cold begins historically with Hippocrates, who recognized that snow and ice were beneficial following soft-tissue injury. In addition, there is a consensus by most clinicians that cold is a standard treatment in soft-tissue injury. It is widely used, inexpensive, and has a variety of methods of application. The purpose of this discussion is to examine the objective scientific evidence for the beneficial effects of cold and to develop a rationale for the use of cold for musculoskeletal disorders.

The methods of cold application include ice, such as ice packs, ice-cup massage, or ice immersion baths. Other methods of application include gel refrigerant packs. These packs can be kept in a freezer, used for their cold application, and then reused with subsequent refreezing. They are expensive. Chemical packs are containers that have a mixture of chemicals that when activated produce an endothermic reaction and cold. These have the disadvantage of containing potentially harmful materials. Coolant sprays are useful in specific situations. Finally, electromechanical devices that produce a combination of refrigeration and compression have been recommended for whole extremity use. Later in this discussion, we will consider the relative efficiency of these various methods and their advantages and disadvantages.

Theoretically, cold may be useful as a physical agent because of evidence that it has an impact in the following areas:

- Metabolism

- Circulation

- Inflammation

- Edema

- Pain

- Muscle spasm

- Collagen stiffness

- Temperature

- Certain clinical applications.

Metabolism.—Experimental evidence substantiates the effect of cold on decreasing metabolism. Specifically, it reduces enzymatic function.

Circulation.—The effect of cold on the vascular system is to produce vasoconstriction. This vasoconstriction does not effect the occurrence of hemorrhage in the clinical setting because it usually is not applied quickly enough. However, it may prevent the extension of hematoma formation.

A phenomenon called cold-induced vasodilatation occurs in the periphery (fingers) following cold immersion. However, there is no scientific evidence that this occurs in other parts of the body such as large muscle groups. There is a lessening of the vasoconstriction effect in deeper tissues, but no vasodilatation in large muscle groups.

Inflammation.—None of the studies that have examined the impact of cold on inflammation have been done in acute traumatic models. All the studies followed chemical or surgically induced trauma. There is no information on chronic inflammation, which might correspond to the rehabilitation setting or beyond the 48 hours of acute care. However, based on the acute experimental model, inflammation is delayed by cold application. However, cold does not eliminate the inflammatory response or decrease long-term chronic inflammation.

Edema.—Cold does not prevent swelling from soft-tissue injury in the animal model and, therefore, probably does not in human soft-tissue injury either. There is no objective data on the impact of cold on permeability at the cellular level. Cold is often used with compression and elevation to prevent swelling. There are no studies that show that the addition of cold is any more effective than compression and elevation alone.

Pain.—Cold produces a decrease in pain by two mechanisms. It blocks sensory transmission of the pain impulse by slowing or eliminating nerve conduction. Second, pain is reduced by decreasing muscle spasm.

Muscle Spasm.—Cold inhibits the stretch reflex and therefore reduces muscle spasm by a direct effect on the muscle spindle.

Collagen Stiffness.—Cold increases collagen stiffness and therefore decreases ligament elasticity and flexibility.

Temperature Effects.—The effects of cold depend upon the temperature of the applied agent, the duration of its application, the surface area over which it is applied, and the body mass to which the cold is applied. All of the preceding factors effect the depth of penetration of the decrease in temperature. Rewarming the cold part depends upon the mass of that body part. For example, a digit will rewarm faster than the forearm.

Based on this information, scientific evidence supports the decrease in skin temperature and subcutaneous tissues with a decrease in muscle temperature up to a depth of 4 cm. No information could be found to support cooling at greater depths.

There were no recent scientific data to explain the redness of the skin that is noted with cold application. There were several controversial reports that this was part of the cold-induced vasodilatation response.

Effects in Clinical Situations.—Experimental evidence supports the concept that cold is superior when used immediately on a soft-tissue injury much as an ankle sprain. Cold does not reduce muscle soreness in the athletic population and the scientific evidence that is available does not support its use before physical activity. Clinical studies recommend the use of cold in therapeutic exercises because the application of cold seems to reduce pain and muscle spasm. The effects of cryokinetics and cryostretch in the rehabilitation phase of soft-tissue injury treatment utilize this approach.

Indications

Based on scientific information, the indications for use of cold should include the acute treatment of soft-tissue injury, within the first 48 hours. Cold decreases metabolism and relieves pain. Secondly, cold is indicated for pain relief in both the acute and chronic phase of musculoskeletal injury. This pain relief is mediated both by decreased muscle spasm and direct decrease in sensory nerve function. Finally, cold is indicated during the rehabilitation phase, i.e., beyond 48 hours, in conjunction with exercise to facilitate mobilization, because it relieves pain by decreasing muscle spasticity, thus allowing the patient to achieve the goal of early motion. However, it is important to recognize that this effect on exercise is for therapeutic exercise alone. Based on the scientific information available, the use of cold should not be extended to sports competition.

Contraindications

Based on the effects of cold, which produce vasoconstriction, decreased metabolism, and decreased neurofunction, and also on certain idiopathic responses, we appreciate that there are some absolute and some relative contraindications to the use of cold.

The *absolute* contraindications are Raynaud's phenomenon, because cold exacerbates this disease; cardiovascular disease, because of an aggravation by pressor response to cold; cryoglobulinemia; and paroxysmal cold hemoglobinuria. Cryoglobulinemia produces chills and fever, and can seriously affect both vision and hearing. The patient may have conjunctival hemorrhage, epistaxis, anemic itching, purpura, and cutaneous ulcerations. These syndromes occur in the presence of associated diseases like lupus erythematosus, vasculitis, multiple myeloma, rheumatoid arthritis, and progressive scleroderma. Paroxysmal cold hemoglobinuria is a hypersensitive phenomenon manifested by malaise, chills, and fever with significant anemia.

The *relative* contraindications are cold allergy, because cold reduces local metabolic rates and blood supply and may slow wound healing; anesthetic skin because of possible frostbite; pheochromocytoma because of aggravation of pressor response; and an arthritic condition.

Clinical Applications

Scientific evidence shows that ice in its various forms is the most efficient and effective method of cold application followed in descending order of effectiveness and efficiency by gel packs, chemical packs, and refrigeration compression machines. Coolant sprays have even more limited application because of the localized effect. Therefore, as long as refrigeration or a cooler is available for transport, ice is the best method of cold application. Gel packs and chemical packs are expensive and not as effective; leaks from these packs may cause burns. Although the refrigerant compression machines may provide an accurate temperature control, there is no scientific evidence to support their being more effective than ice alone.

Sprays such as ethyl chloride are useful for local injection because of their circumscribed anesthetic effect. However, there is significant risk with improper use, which includes burn and frostbite.

Although the optimal temperature from experimental information seems to be between 10 and 18°C, it should be noted that experimental work indicates that ice from the freezer has a temperature between -5 and 0°C, and a cold whirlpool from 4 to 15°C, and a slush bath from 0 to 4°C. These temperatures all seem to be much colder than necessary for the therapeutic effects necessary from cold. Some consideration needs to be given to the careful evaluation of the soft tissues with these various methods of application and means of accurately controlling the temperature.

Some other areas of caution include using cold alone or with pressure over nerves such as the ulnar or peroneal nerve and the risk of neuropraxia. In addition, cold should not be used as a method of pain relief before sports activity because of its effect of collagen stiffness and reduction in flexibility, which may lead to further injury.

Summary

The consensus of the panel on cold was (1) cold has a beneficial effect in soft-tissue injury; (2) the benefit is primarily in the first 48 hours following trauma or surgery; (3) cold has a later value during rehabilitation to facilitate mobilization through relief of pain and muscle spasm; (4) information is insufficient to support use of cold to reduce inflammation in chronic inflammatory conditions. Based on the scientific information available to us, we support the principles of heat before exercise or physical activity including sports, and ice for soft-tissue injuries.

COLD MODALITIES: RECOMMENDATIONS FOR FURTHER RESEARCH

We recommend that scientific research be conducted to standardize the methods for applications of cold by determining the effects of various methods of cold application on the skin and deeper tissue temperatures.

- To determine the cause of skin redness after cold application.

- To determine if cold is useful in treating other forms of muscular spasticity such as neuromuscular disorders.

- To evaluate the relative value of ice plus compression and elevation vs. compression and elevation alone or ice alone on soft-tissue injury.

- To create a model of traumatic inflammation to evaluate the effect of cold. (Current information is all based on surgically and chemically induced inflammation. We need a model to study the effects of cold on hemorrhage, tissue permeability, and inflammation.)

3

Electrical Modalities

Kenneth Singer, M.D.

Robert D'Ambrosia, M.D.

Ben Graf, M.D.

George (Kim) Hewson, M.D.

Robert Hunter, M.D.

William Stanish, M.D.

ELECTRICAL MODALITIES IN SPORTS MEDICINE

The use of electrostimulation modalities in sports medicine has flourished during the past decade. The charge to this committee was to gather and synthesize information that would assist the sports medicine clinician to better understand the proper place of this modality in the treatment of patients. This has been accomplished by reviewing the extensive available literature regarding this entity. In reaching its conclusions, the committee attempted to weigh more heavily those works that were considered to have the higher scientific validity. While the committee attempted to evaluate the modalities, no attempt was made to evaluate specific devices or specific manufacturers.

The use of electricity in medicine is not new. Scribonius Largus, a Roman physician, described the use of electric eels, rays, and torpedo fish in the treatment of gout and headaches. He brought the affected part into direct contact with the electric animal in a bucket of water, and the irritated ray emitted a retaliatory jolt and stunned the area, often relieving the pain for several hours, according to reports. In the 1850s hand-cranked transcutaneous electrical neurologic stimulation (TENS) units were used for the relief of pain. Between 1900 and 1940, numerous units were marketed that were essentially battery-operated faradic devices used for "bath, massage, and douche." There is no evidence of controlled studies correlating with these alleged results. In the early part of this century, electric devices were manufactured and promoted for treating acne, abscesses, alopecia, anemia, asthma, constipation, corns, goiter, gout, headaches, hemorrhoids, lumbago, urinary incontinence, shingles, and, many other ailments.

In 1965 Melzack and Wall first postulated their "gate theory" of pain control, which attempted in a scientific way to explain why electrical stimulation was effective in pain relief, and that explanation provided the emphasis for more widespread use of electrical devices in the control of pain.

All is still not science. We are looking for simple ways to solve problems, but the solutions remain elusive.

Principles of Electricity

A brief description of the electrical principles pertinent to these devices is appropriate. The monograph by Prentice (1986) describes the concepts of electricity as they apply to biologic behavior, and the reader should refer to that reference for more details.

Electric devices can put out either alternating current, such as that found in common household electricity, or direct current, which is like that produced by a battery. Alternating current can have different waveforms, e.g., square or sinusoidal, or spiked and intermittent, and so forth. Similarly, direct current, also known as galvanic current, can be continuous or intermittent, and can also have different waveforms. Keep in mind that it is the OUTPUT of the electrical device that is important, and not what powers it. Whether the device is powered by batteries or a wall socket does not matter; the electronics of the device can alter the source of power to produce whatever type of electricity (alternating or direct), waveform (square, sinusoidal, spiked, etc), frequency (continuous, modulated, etc) is desired.

The frequency, the amplitude, and the waveform of the output can be varied. The frequency is the number of cycles or pulses per second, usually referred to as cps, or hertz (Hz). The amplitude is the strength of the pulse. Either the frequency or the amplitude can be continuous or variable, which is called modulated. The waveform may be varied in any number of ways. The specifications of any device will usually give in diagrammatic form the stimulation parameters.

Three specific clinical applications of electrical devices were examined by the committee. Specifically, these were the use of electric modalities (1) to relieve pain, (2) to increase muscle strength, and (3) to promote soft-tissue healing. Because not enough information is available on the use of electric modalities for soft-tissue healing, we will discuss herein only pain control and muscle strengthening.

Pain Control—TENS

Transcutaneous electric nerve stimulation is usually defined as the application of an electrical current through the skin to a peripheral nerve or nerves for the control of pain. The transcutaneous electric nerve stimulators are widely used in everyday practice.

Mechanism of Action.—Two basic theories explain why electric stimulation can alter pain perception.

In 1965, Melzack and Wall postulated the gate control theory of pain relief, which first gave credence to the idea that cutaneous stimulation could alter the perception of pain. Pain sensation is carried to the spinal cord by small slow unmyelinated nerve fibers. Light touch and proprioception sensations are carried by way of myelinated fast larger fibers. The gate theory postulates that if the larger, more easily excited sensory fibers are overstimulated, they can flood the pathways to the brain and close the gate to transmission of pain fibers, thereby diminishing awareness of painful stimuli. When the external stimulation has ceased, unless there is an accommodation to the electrical stimulus, the "gate" is then open and pain perception returns.

The second theory that explains the efficacy of TENS is based on the existence of natural opiates. Electric stimulation of sensory nerves stimulates the release of opiates, namely beta-endorphins produced by the pituitary gland and enkephalins, which emanate from the spinal cord. Both of these substances will decrease pain perception.

Stimulation of sensory nerves with frequencies in the 70-Hz range, referred to as high-frequency TENS, will increase the pain threshold, but does not stimulate the release of endorphins, thereby implicating the gate control theory. However, stimulation with lower frequencies will cause pain relief, which can be blocked by the administration of opiate antagonists, thereby implicating the stimulation of endorphins release as its mechanism of action. Low-frequency TENS is sometimes likened to acupuncture. Therefore, from a theoretical point of view, a TENS unit that uses either high or low frequencies would seem to be effective in controlling pain under varying circumstances.

The experimental evidence is not quite so clear. Direct low-frequency electrical stimulation of certain areas may produce significant elevation of endorphin levels in the human cerebrospinal fluid and thereby block pain perception. Beta-endorphins, probably the most potent endogenous opiate, are 30 times more potent on a molar basis than morphine.

Sjolund and Eriksson (1979) administered naloxone, an opiate antagonist, and sterile saline to patients in a double-blind study in order to test the role of the endorphins and enkephalins. These results indicate that low-frequency TENS utilized endorphins, whereas high-frequency TENS employed some other mechanism. O'Brien et al. (1984) were unable to measure a significant change in the blood concentrations of beta-endorphins following the use of TENS regardless of the frequency and were unable to reverse the effect of TENS analgesia by naloxone injections.

Clinical Studies of Effectiveness of TENS.—The numerous studies of the efficacy of TENS are difficult to evaluate, as it is difficult, if not impossible, to design a truly double-blind study. Therefore, many of the results must attempt to quantify, either directly or indirectly, the perception of pain, a task that at best is difficult, and at worst impossible.

Subjective testimony as to the effectiveness of any treatment or medication that attempts to relieve pain is flawed by the well-described placebo effect. Most studies evaluating pain relief fail to take into account the placebo effect, which can be responsible for up to 30% of pain relief. The placebo effect is maximal when applied directly to the site of pain, and often decreases with time. Both of these factors are characteristic of the use of TENS units.

By way of objective evaluation, there are several studies that seem to show that TENS units are effective in pain relief, by decreasing narcotics needed, length of hospital stay after arthrotomy, and the mobilization time after surgery. Arvidsson and Eriksson (1986) objectively tested the results of high-frequency TENS to assess pain and showed that placebo TENS had no significant effect on pain perception or IEMG, while high-frequency TENS decreased pain perception by 50%

at rest and by 11% after quadriceps contraction. Jenson et al. (1985) showed that a group of patients treated with TENS following arthroscopic surgery experienced less pain and required less narcotics and regained strength quicker than the control group or the placebo group, and Smith et al. (1983) showed that hospital stays were decreased following arthrotomy when TENS was used. Transcutaneous electric nerve stimulation has been effective in treating patients with patella femoral pain and adhesive capsulitis, apparently by decreasing pain sufficiently to allow better compliance with muscle strengthening or range and motion exercise programs. However, several studies that seem equally good show that TENS is not effective when evaluating the same parameters, so the results are not conclusive.

There are many reports describing pain control in a variety of other orthopedic conditions, but the data are primarily subjective and little objective data were noted in our research of the literature.

Therefore, from evaluation of the literature, it appears that treatment of early postoperative pain or pain from acute injuries responds to TENS to some degree in some persons, but with a variable and often unpredictable response.

Numerous articles claim that TENS controls pain in a variety of chronic conditions, but they produce no objective data. Most of these reports are deficient and show that pain grading techniques are extremely difficult to design and interpret.

Use of TENS.—For TENS to be effective, electrode placement must be appropriate. Effective stimulation can occur over the peripheral nerve, the dermatome, and at trigger points, but is usually best when situated over the area of maximal pain. The most effective site for stimulation can be determined empirically, and most physical therapists will be able to select the correct placement site.

Electrode contact with the skin is important. There

are different types of electrodes. Some are held on with straps, and others, such as those used with portable units, are usually held to the skin with adhesives and changed every 2 to 4 days. One method uses suction cups to apply the stimulus to the skin. While electrode placement site is important, it is unlikely that the type of electrode is particularly important in the outcome.

The effectiveness of TENS will vary with alteration of the stimulation. As the frequency and amplitude of stimulation increases, up to the level of discomfort, the effect on pain relief also increases, such as in treatment of adhesive capsulitis of the shoulder, where TENS has been used to reduce pain so that exercises can be tolerated.

Indications and Contraindications.—The indications, best supported in the literature for the use of TENS to reduce pain, seem to be applicable in the immediate postsurgical or postinjury situation. Most observers note that TENS is less effective as the time from injury or surgery increases, and also that the effectiveness seems to decrease with time of use. It is sometimes used in chronic pain conditions, but the evidence for its effectiveness is lacking.

There are few contraindications for TENS use. It should not be used in persons with pacemakers, stimulation should not be applied over the carotid sinus, and it should probably not be used during pregnancy, as the effects are unknown.

There are also certain situations in which TENS, while not contraindicated, appears to be predictably associated with a poor response. Individuals with psychogenic pain do not respond to TENS. Drug-experienced individuals experiencing pain from any cause seem not to respond well, and the drug experience may even be as limited as the use of narcotics for pain relief after surgery. This has been postulated as a possible reason to explain the extreme variability of response to TENS under what would seem to be standard criteria. Patients with wound drainage even in the absence of infection seem less likely to respond than patients with dry wounds. And lastly, improper electrode placement will not be associated with a good response.

Cost.—At present, the purchase cost of a portable TENS unit is in the range of $550 to $700, and it can usually be rented for approximately $85 monthly. Costs incurred during inpatient usage will depend on whether the patient controls the unit or whether the therapist uses TENS as a treatment modality.

Comment.—Transcutaneous electric nerve stimulation units can be effective in the control of pain in some persons and in some conditions. The response is variable and unpredictable; there are few complications and few contraindications. The results are usually not long-lasting, and it is often difficult on evaluation to determine how much of the result is related to the placebo effect. It is important to have somebody who is familiar with the device and with its use to instruct the patient. Perhaps the most effective use of TENS would be in moderating pain sufficiently to allow better compliance with specific exercise programs. Whether or not it is cost-effective must be determined on an individual basis.

Much additional research is needed in order to determine the proper role of TENS in the treatment of pain. The development of a good model that will allow double-blind testing is particularly important, and after the model is available, the effectiveness of TENS can be proved or disproved. The modality can then be fine-tuned by studying the other variables, such as the stimulus, the optimal time of use, and comparisons among the various TENS units now available.

Pain Control—Other Devices

Neuroprobe.—The neuroprobe is a type of electric stimulation unit that can be used to search out tender areas or trigger points, and may be effective in reducing pain. It may also be used for locating the ideal sites for electrode placement for the conventional TENS unit.

Interferential Unit.—Another type of stimulation sometimes used to control pain is the interferential unit. Electric signals from two sets of electrodes with the same waveform are applied so that they arrive at the point to be stimulated from two different directions. The area where the current overlaps is called the interference pattern, and the intensity summates in a manner that can be effective in modifying pain.

Muscle Strength Gains—Electrical Stimulation

The possible use of electrical stimulation to increase muscle strength is appealing. Evaluation of strength enhancement must be considered in two completely separate settings—one, strengthening a weakened muscle, and the other, the possibility of enhancing the strength of a normal muscle.

Increasing the strength of a muscle can be accomplished by repeated maximal or submaximal contraction of that muscle. There exists a high degree of specificity in strength enhancement, such that when a muscle is trained isometrically, it responds isometrically, and when trained isokinetically, for all practical purposes only isokinetic strength increases occur. This principle of training specificity is quite predictable, and it is therefore necessary to measure strength gains with that specificity in mind.

The rationale behind the strength enhancement is that electrical stimulation can either increase the maximum contractile force in the muscle, or that it can recruit more fibers to contract with a given stimulus, thereby enhancing the strength of that contraction. If any strength enhancement is to occur, the electrical stimulation must produce a strong tetanic contraction.

Electric stimulation is achieved by stimulating the motor nerve to a muscle by means of electrodes placed on the skin. While there has been some work with isotonic and isokinetic strengthening with electrical stimulation, most of the work has been done with electric stimulation in the isometric mode.

A persistent problem that emerges when one attempts to evaluate the effectiveness of electrical stimulation to improve strength is the lack of standardization of the stimulus. The stimulus variables are frequency, duration, pulse shape, intensity, and charge. To date there are no studies that interrelate these variables to compare their effectiveness in inducing effective strength-improving muscle contractions.

Most stimulators commercially available produce either a biphasic (alternating) current or monophasic pulsating (direct) output (EGS). However, studies relating the variables of stimuli such as frequency, modulation, pulse shape and duration, and amplitude, are lacking, so it is not possible at this time to compare the wide variety of stimulators now in use. As an example, reports vary as to the best method of stimulation to activate muscle contraction by motor nerves. However, despite the many electrical stimulators now available, there have been no demonstrable differences among them in their ability to induce muscle contractions.

The pulse frequency is considered to be particularly important. It requires 20 Hz or more to begin to achieve tetany. Low-frequency stimulators are usually in the 50-Hz range, and medium frequencies are in the range of 100-to 10,000-Hz range. Stimulation with frequencies above 5,000 is much more comfortable, and that has given rise to medium-range stimulator frequencies. However, in many instances it is only the carrier signal that has higher frequency, while the actual stimulation frequency is 50 Hz. As Lloyd et al. (1986) indicated, since the maximum firing frequency during a maximum voluntary contraction is less than 100 Hz, "...the rationale for using stimulation far in excess of this figure has yet to be established."

Various investigators have looked at electrical muscle stimulation (EMS)-induced force and torque production, and, while the results vary somewhat from study to study, there do not seem to be appreciable differences in the different stimulators tested.

Strength Gains in Abnormal Muscles.—There are many studies indicating that the loss of strength normally accompanying limb injury, immobilization, or surgery may be significantly retarded by EMS. Eriksson and Haggmark (1979) showed better muscle function in a group of patients after reconstruction of the ACL when treated with EMS and exercise, than with exercise alone. However, the preponderance of evidence available to date seems to indicate that EMS and voluntary exercise are equally effective in retarding strength loss or increasing strength gains in abnormal muscles.

In the rehabilitation setting, evidence suggests that EMS may retard muscle strength loss and increase muscle strength, and when used in conjunction with voluntary exercise, may be more effective in increasing muscle strength. This presupposes a muscle that is partially denervated either because of injury, surgery, or disuse from immobilization. The factors seem to be the same in the partially denervated muscle or that subjected to disuse. It is generally agreed that EMS is effective in maintaining and improving muscle strength in weakened musculature, but how much more effective it is in relation to voluntary exercise cannot be conclusively stated. It may be that the benefits are a result of its reeducation role in facilitating early voluntary muscle contraction, and, perhaps, also pain relief. Eriksson's studies seem to indicate that EMS is sometimes more beneficial after surgery, but clearly more so in women, and probably not in men. The study of strength loss as a result of immobilization by Morrissey et al. (1985) showed that muscle stimulation can decrease strength loss that occurs as a result of immobilization at 6 weeks, but when examined after 12 weeks, or 6 weeks after immobilization was discontinued, the strength losses were identical for the stimulated and nonstimulated group. They also showed, as have many others, that stimulation does not increase the girth of the leg, and that stimulation seemed to have no effect on the pain that occurred during maximal quadriceps contraction.

Another study showed that when strength was measured at the seventh to ninth week following surgery, no significant difference existed between the strength of those patients treated with EMS and exercise and those treated with exercise alone. adding the EMS did not make an appreciable difference.

Yet, certainly electrical stimulation of muscle has some effects. Stanish et al. (1982) and Eriksson et al. (1981) have shown that the biochemical changes occurring in the muscles of immobilized limbs are retarded by EMS. Just how this translates into data that can be applied and be clinically effective remains elusive.

The argument is made by the advocates and manufacturers of EMS (and TENS) that they should be used early following surgery or injury to prevent the early atrophy and loss of strength until more active exercise programs can be introduced. There is perhaps merit in this approach; yet no studies that look at the long-term effects indicate that long-lasting benefits accrue under those circumstances.

If in order to improve strength, maximal or nearly maximal contractions must occur to the point of fatigue, then it must be necessary for EMS to be able to accomplish this. Review of the available information seems to indicate that maximum contractile forces can be produced by voluntary contractions as well or better than produced by electrical stimulation, with a few exceptions.

Research in the area of strengthening weakened muscles is badly needed. The optimal stimulus variables (pulse shape, charge, duration, frequency, and intensity) that are required to produce the desired motor response need to be established. At the present time there are no systematic studies that relate all of the characteristics of the stimulus to force production in different muscles. For example, at the present time no consistent differences have been demonstrated between the ability of monophasic or pulsating direct current or biphasic or alternating outputs to induce muscle contraction. Each type of current possibly has its advantages and disadvantages, but these have yet to be demonstrated.

Strengthening Normal Muscles.—The use of electrical stimulation to enhance the strength of normal muscles is a relatively new concept. It originates from claims made by a scientist from the Soviet Union named Kotts, who reported at a 1977 Canadian symposium at Concordia University that a specific stimulation program was able to increase strength in normal muscles significantly. His program consisted of using 2,500 cps frequency current alternating 10-msec bursts with 10 msec of rest. He used a duty cycle consisting of 10 seconds of stimulation to the muscle followed by 50 seconds of rest. He stated that with only 3 weeks of this program, major gains were achieved in strength and endurance, a decrease in subcutaneous fat, and increased limb girth. However, despite numerous attempts, no study in the Western bloc has been able to reproduce these data.

There is general agreement in the literature that EMS alone can increase the strength of a normal muscle when used in a variety of experimental protocols. However, it has not been demonstrated that EMS, whether used alone or combined with an exercise program, is any more effective in enhancing strength than a good voluntary exercise program.

Application of Muscle Stimulation.—The application of muscle stimulation is straightforward. The electrodes are placed such that stimulation can reach the motor nerve to the muscle involved, and since the electricity will travel through tissue, the exact placement site is not critical. The frequency and amplitude of the stimulus are increased until a tetanic contraction can be obtained without significant discomfort.

How long and how often the stimulation should be applied is controversial, but probably 7- to 10-second stimulations are needed many times throughout the day. Formerly, it was thought that the more the stimulation, the more the gain in strength, but more recent evidence indicates that strength gains may not accrue even with long periods of stimulation.

If a TENS unit was used, and the electrodes were placed over the motor nerve, the same effect would be obtained if the stimulating current were increased. While there may be many variations in the output of the electric device, such as frequency, amplitude, and waveform, it appears that the body has difficulty distinguishing them; electricity is electricity, whether it originates from a TENS unit, a muscle-stimulating unit, or a spark plug; the principles are the same despite the variations.

It is clear that since exercise is probably at least as effective as muscle stimulation, if not more, the person should be on an active exercise program along with the stimulation.

Indications.—The indications for the use of electrical stimulation are controversial. At present, the only reasonable use is to increase strength in a muscle that has been weakened, denervated, or possibly immobilized, but the constraints and limitations, as noted in the preceding paragraphs, should be kept in mind. Based on available information, there is probably not a good reason to use electrical stimulation routinely.

Contraindications.—The contraindications for the use of electrical stimulation are the same as those of TENS, and the complications are essentially nonexistent. The main contraindication is the lack of proven effectiveness.

Cost.—The cost of using electrical stimulation will vary depending upon how it is used, the geographical region where the treatment occurs, and whether it is on an inpatient or outpatient basis. Inpatient treatment with the high-voltage galvanic unit, for example, will cost approximately $30 per treatment when administered by a physical therapist, while the use of a portable device, such as the Respond unit, will cost approximately $20 as a set-up charge and $10 to $20 daily. For outpatient use, the Respond unit is representative of the many units available, and its cost is approximately $950 to purchase the unit or $75 to $90 monthly if rented.

Effectiveness.—In summary, there does seem to be evidence, although not conclusive, that electrical stimulation can increase strength in muscles that are weakened by injury or disuse. It appears that the effect is not long-lasting, and that it may well not be better than gains that could be produced by a good exercise program. Data suggest that electrical stimulation may be suited to the initial management of motor reeducation, as active exercise is the eventual objective in rehabilitation programs. There is no good reproducible evidence that electrical stimulation of muscles is as effective as a training modality to increase strength in normal muscles.

Summary

As is the case with all modalities in sports medicine, electric stimulation does not offer any magical solutions. Electric stimulation to control pain certainly has some applications, while the role of strengthening of muscles with electric stimulation is less clear based upon the available literature. This is another area in medicine where randomized prospective evaluation of these forms of treatment would have been of great value before they become so widely established into therapeutic practice. There is so much testimonial and anecdotal support for the use of these modalities, that as clinicians we must be particularly vigilant and attempt to separate the science from the marketing strategy.

The consensus of the panel on electrical modalities was:

- Electric stimulation as a modality to modify pain perception is effective in some individuals and should be considered as a therapeutic modality to be tried when pain limits function or additional therapy.

- Electric stimulation may be useful to improve strength in muscles weakened by surgery or in-

GRIMSBY COLLEGE LIBRARY

jury where maximal voluntary contraction is not possible.

- Electric stimulation to improve strength in normal muscles is not warranted based upon currently available information.

- There is too little information available to determine whether the use of electricity to hasten the healing of soft-tissue injury is effective.

ELECTRICAL MODALITIES RECOMMENDATIONS FOR FURTHER RESEARCH

Research opportunities abound in the area of electrical stimulation. Effective research is presently hindered by the lack of available machinery to provide double-blind studies, the difficulty in quantitating injuries in order to select for comparison groups of similar injuries, and the problems inherent in using and quantitating pain as an endpoint and comparing pain in different individuals.

We recommend that scientific research be conducted:

- To create a device that looks and feels the same as the electric stimulators available in order to perform double-blind studies.

- To examine the effectiveness of TENS by using double-blind techniques and equivalent injuries with a simple and reproducible pain-grading scale.

- To create experiments that will identify the effect of varying the stimulation parameters in TENS and EMS units.

- To encourage research laboratories to investigate the morphologic (electron microscopic) and histochemical changes that occur with electrical stimulation of muscle.

4 | Therapeutic Exercise Modalities

Jesse DeLee, M.D.

Fred Allman, M.D.

James Howe, M.D.

Lonnie Paulos, M.D.

Ed Wojtys, M.D.

William Woods, M.D.

GLOSSARY TERMS FOR THERAPEUTIC EXERCISE

Static contraction—a muscle contraction that is not associated with any joint motion.

Dynamic contraction—a muscle contraction associated with joint motion.

Isometric contraction—a static contraction in which the muscle maintains a constant length.

Isotonic contraction—a dynamic muscle contraction against a constant or variable resistance in which there is a change of length of the muscle, either concentric or eccentric.

- *Eccentric (negative) contraction*—muscle contraction in which the muscle lengthens while contracting.

- *Concentric (positive) Contraction*—muscle contraction in which the muscle shortens as a result of the contraction.

- *Constant resistance exercise*—an exercise done with unchanging resistance such that the muscle contracts differing percentages of its maximum throughout the range of motion.

- *Variable resistance exercise*—exercise in which the resistance is varied, i.e., by use of lever arms or cams, so as to approximate the strength of an individual muscle.

Isokinetic contractions—contraction against an accommodating resistance at a preset constant speed.

- *Accommodating resistance*—is the resistance applied in isokinetic exercise in which the speed of movement is controlled so that the resistance supplied is in proportion to the force generated by the muscle at each point throughout its range motion.

Strength—maximum force generated by a muscle contraction without relation to time.

Endurance—ability to persist in physical activity, to resist muscular fatigue. There are two major components involved in measuring endurance:

- *Local or muscular endurance*—duration of contraction, which is limited by a finite energy supply or the buildup of acid metabolic end products. (Energy stores are concluded due to pressure of the contracted muscle.)

- *General or circulorespiratory endurance*—ability of the physiological and psychological systems to resist fatigue in gross body activity. The physiological factors include respiration, circulation, heat dissipation, nervous system, homeostatic mechanisms, and peripheral muscle function. The two most important physiological factors are oxygen transport and metabolic capacity of the muscle involved.

Training effect—improvement in test performance based solely on familiarity with testing techniques.

Proprioceptive neuromuscular facilitation—technique that facilitates motor performance by stimulating joint proprioceptors by strength and applied resistance through a functional muscle pattern. Proprioceptive neuromuscular facilitation is a flexibility trauma technique that uses the normal neurological passive stretch, active contact, relaxed pattern. The mechanism may be by autogenic inhibition and active mobilization of connective tissue.

Robotics—active dynamometers with direct drive mechanics capable of moving a limb throughout a range of motion, the parameters being controlled by a computer or electronics.

Power—product of force and distance over which the force is applied divided by the time during which the force is applied. It is the time rate at which work is performed or energy expended. Work or energy, over time, equals watts (joules per second).

Hypertrophy—enlargement of muscle fibers accompanied by increased muscle strength.

Torque—product of force times the lever arm.

Lever arm—perpendicular distance from the axis of rotation to the line of action of the force.

PRINCIPLES OF REHABILITATION

In treating athletes, be they football players, basketball players, baseball players, soccer players, or even those engaged in recreational sports such as skiing, golf, and tennis, no phases of treatment are more important than conditioning and rehabilitation. The effectiveness of rehabilitation in the recovery period, either after injury or after a surgical procedure, will usually determine the degree and success of future athletic competition. As sports medicine physicians, we recognize that injuries sustained during athletic participation are usually produced by circumstances inherent in respective athletic performance. Recurrent identical trauma is likely if the athlete continues to participate in that sport. A variety of programs and equipment for rehabilitation has been used since DeLorme introduced the progressive resistive exercise routine during World War II. During this same 40 years, considerable progress has been made in other aspects of sports medicine as well.

Five years later (1950), O'Donoghue first advocated early surgical repair for torn knee ligaments. Innovations have also been made in protective equipment and playing facilities, and the certification of athletic trainers has become a reality. Most important of all, however, has been the development of a greater awareness by coaches and trainers, as well as physicians, of the need for prompt proper medical care for all injured athletes, and which, of course, includes the need for total rehabilitation following injury. During the last 30 years, there has been an increased participation and emphasis on sports at all levels with an increased tempo in these sports.

Goal of Rehabilitation

Injuries sustained during athletic participation are usually produced by circumstances inherent in athletic performance. They are characterized by exposure to recurrent identical trauma, making reinjury likely. Too often the physician, trainer, or physical therapist fails to take this point into consideration when supervising rehabilitation. As a result, the end point of treatment is often far short of a safe performance level. The best protection is balanced bilateral muscular strength as well as antagonist muscle balance. The goal of treatment must be restoration of function to the greatest possible degree and in the shortest possible time, although time must be allowed for maturation of damaged tissue.

The SAID Principle

In conditioning or reconditioning for vigorous sports activity following injury, it is necessary to understand the SAID principle, or specific adaptation in imposed demands. Simply stated, the training program must attempt to adapt the individual to the demands that may be made upon him or her during athletic performance. Adaptation is specific and refers to the alteration of the structure or function of an organ or part as a result of an altered environment. Function increases with use; functions we do not use, we lose. The intensity, duration, and frequency of activity are all related to the functional capacity that is developed. Unfortunately, today's youth, because of relative inactivity, do not have sufficient exposure to vigorous activity, and are, therefore, poorly adapted to the environment created by certain sports, especially contact sports. The result has been a gradual progressive increase in the frequency and severity of injuries, especially knee injuries, and a high incidence of reinjury—the reinjury being related not only to poor adaptation over many years but also to failure in ability to restore normal function.

The athlete with ligamentous laxity is far more susceptible to injury than the athlete without such laxity. The stretch effect of a normal ligament is proprioceptive in nature and results in a stimulation to the surrounding musculature that calls the muscle into supportive function of the joint. The muscular action stabilizes the joint and thus defends the ligaments against abnormal stress. A strong musculature causes the joint to be more firmly bound together and thus reduces abnormal movement. A joint is a torque-transmitting mechanism, and if it is called upon to transmit a force that exceeds its capacity, then damage to the joint or its surrounding soft tissue may occur. In attempting to restore muscle function, therefore, it is important not to overstress the joint beyond its capable range.

Rehabilitation of the athlete with an injury deals primarily with restoration of muscle and joint function. The assurance given the athlete that his or her muscular strength and functional capacity are at a high level of supportive quality is a physiological as well as a psychological necessity in order for him or her to return to the field of competition. Haphazard unproven methods of rehabilitation are usually ineffective and fall far short of the desired goal. Practice for the event itself does not make sufficient demands upon all of the physiological systems supporting the performance. The performer must therefore supplement practice of the event with artificial exercise designed to develop supporting physiological mechanisms to the point that they can make a maximum contribution to the overall effort.

Individualized Rehabilitation

Rehabilitation of the injured athlete must be individualized. No single exercise or piece of apparatus known to science today can be classified as a panacea;

likewise, while elaborate and extensive tables and gadgets are available, and frequently desirable, proven methods may be used that require little or no special equipment. Disabled persons must rehabilitate themselves, but they must be given proper guidance and evaluation if they are to succeed.

Types of Therapeutic Exercise

Therapeutic exercise is defined as bodily movements prescribed to restore or alter favorably specific functions in an individual following an injury. They may be active or passive. *Active exercise* is purposeful voluntary motion that is performed by the person himself, without resistance, and with or without the aid of gravity. Active exercise may be static, kinetic, or isokinetic. *Static exercise* is that which is performed without producing joint movement. The contracting muscle shortens, producing the movement, which is an *isotonic exercise*. Isokinetic exercises are those in which joint motion occurs at a controlled rate. *Concentric contraction* occurs when a muscle is contracted from the extended to the shortened position. *Eccentric contraction* occurs when the tensed muscle lengthens. An example of a concentric contraction would be flexion of the elbow in performing a pullup. An example of an eccentric contraction is that of slowly lowering the body into the extended position from the flexed position after doing a pullup, since the muscle is maintaining tension while actually lengthening. *Passive exercises* are those performed for the injured athlete by another person or by a mechanical appliance. Passive exercise is carried out by the application of some external force with minimal participation of the muscle action by the injured athlete. It may be forced or nonforced. The nonforced exercises are those used to help maintain normal joint motion and are kept within a painless range of motion, for the most part, while forced passive exercises are those that usually produced movement beyond the limits of the free range of motion and are often associated with some discomfort to the patient.

Rehabilitation as a Team Approach

Rehabilitation of the injured athlete should be a team approach involving not only the injured athlete, but also the team physician, trainer, the orthopedic surgeon, and the physical therapist. If the injured athlete rehabilitation program is to succeed, all of the aforementioned individuals are important in making certain that the exercise prescription is formulated properly and carried out correctly.

Formulating an Exercise Prescription

Normal muscle and joint function is restored by a training program. A prescription for a training program must include the exercise to be prescribed, the precautions, the duration and intensity of the exercise, and the nature and range of the exercise movement, as well as the rhythm, timing, and proper progression order to achieve maximum performance in the shortest possible time. The objectives of training are the development of muscle strength and endurance, flexibility, the ability to yield to passive stretch and to relax, and neuromuscular reeducation.

The Exercise.—Three main factors must be considered in prescribing the exercise: the purpose of the exercise, how it is to be administered, and its relationship to other exercises that may be prescribed. Proper selection of an exercise must be based on knowledge of the principles of joint dynamics; also, the exercise must be able to fulfill its designed purpose. The proper execution of an exercise is extremely important. Failure to achieve the desired benefits usually indicates poor selection of the exercise. Injury may occur if the exercise is not properly executed.

Precautions.—The precautions should include care for any existing conditions that might alter the response of the person to the exercise program. Exercise must be administered within the limits imposed by the existing status of the individual. The kinetic hazards imposed by the exercise must also be considered. The athlete with chondromalacia of the patella should avoid exercises that include range of motion with weight initially. Even later in the rehabilitation program, when range of motion exercises are added to the routine, it is better to use an isokinetic type of exercise, or an isometric exercise, rather than an isotonic exercise.

SAID Principle.—It is extremely important in prescribing the exercise that the future plans of the athlete be known. What are his desires for future participation? If it is for a sport such as football, higher performance levels should be sought than for the individual who seeks to play golf, archery, or any one of the other noncontact type sports.

Duration.—The duration of each exercise period and of the total amount of time required for the program must be considered. The duration may vary from only a few days following a contusion to a period of months following multiple ligamentous injuries, which constitute a major disability.

Intensity.—The intensity will vary according to the extent of the injury for which the exercise prescription is being ordered. For minor injuries, the intensity may be great initially and duration short, while, in a more severely injured athlete, the intensity will be low initially. Intensity of exercise regulates growth stimulation in muscle, and growth stimulation relates almost directly to strength gain. Factors that must be considered in the intensity of exercise include the resistance load and the range of motion, to indicate the distance that the load is moved, the speed of movement, and the duration of the activity.

Nature of the Movement.—The nature of the movement is characterized by its speed, the method of loading as it effects joint dynamics, and whether or not it is performed unilaterally or bilaterally, either simultaneously or alternately. The length of the lever arm, the attachment points of muscles and tendons, and their angles of insertion are important in determining these characteristics.

Range of the Movement.—The range of movement is determined by the distance the body part covers in exercise. Immediately following injury, or following surgery, an exercise might be prescribed without any movement of the involved joint, whereas, as improvement takes place, the range of movement will be gradually increased in the recovery period, the range of motion should be as complete as possible. The best results in restoring full muscle function are achieved when the muscles are contracted throughout the entire range of motion of the joints involved.

Rhythm.—The rhythm relates not only to that which is carried out during each movement but also as it relates to other movements. In the initial phases of the rehabilitation program, it is important to teach effort-relaxation cycles so that the muscle does not remain in a state of constant tension. As the exercise program progresses, less emphasis needs to be placed on effort-relaxation cycles as they become more or less subconscious. It has been demonstrated that a resting muscle recovers more quickly if it is exposed to a workload of low intensity during the resting period between heavy exertions. Rhythm in the overall exercise scheme is extremely important because it involves utilization of exercises that effect large muscle groups prior to those that effect the small muscle groups. The greater the mass of involved muscles, the greater the value of the exercise. For example, in a knee rehabilitation program, it would be far better to have exercises involving the hip extensors work first because of the large muscle group that is involved. Secondly, an exercise such as the half knee bend would be prescribed, followed by other more specific exercises, such as knee extension, knee flexion, and, lastly, ankle plantar flexion and dorsiflexion exercises.

Timing.—Timing relates to exposure with a given exercise as well as the time allowed between each exercise. It relates to the coordination of muscle response, and also the states of rehabilitation, whether immediately after injury or late in the rehabilitation program.

Progression.—Progression in a training is essential. It relates to range of motion, load, speed, power, and energy expenditure in relationship to each exercise as well as to the total exercise program. An attempt should be made to produce some sign of progress in each exercise session with the development of power potential the ultimate goal. Muscles must be worked to the point of "momentary failure" or "exhaustion" if a high performance level is to be achieved.

Neuromuscular Reeducation.—Neuromuscular reeducation primarily involves development of a proprioceptive awareness. Correction of posture and the use of passive, active, and resistive movements all seem to be essential to complete proprioceptive response. It is important, therefore, to realize that normal function will, in most cases, return more quickly to the athlete who is allowed to continue with activities that permit near normal function but do not interfere with the normal healing process.

Functional Evaluation

A functional evaluation is necessary to determine whether or not the athlete is ready to return to normal participation. The functional evaluation should be immediately preceded by an evaluation of girth, strength, and goniometric measurements of all adjacent structures in the involved extremity. Even after the athlete has achieved a safe performance level and is allowed to return to full participation, he or she should be recalled for periodic reevaluation at appropriate times. It is only through periodic reevaluation that an athlete can maintain a safe performance level. While many will be able to maintain such a performance level with relative ease, others will have to continue with some form of rehabilitation after their return to activity in order to maintain such a high level.

The primary responsibility for the exercise prescription resides with the treating physician. It therefore is important for the physician to have an understanding of these basic principles as well as their application.

Selection of the modalities to use in carrying out the exercise prescription will be determined by the availability of the modalities as well as the knowledge of the person directly supervising the rehabilitation.

Although certain advantages may be offered by the expensive and more sophisticated equipment, the essential needs can be achieved by a variety of exercises that will incorporate the basic principles.

ISOMETRIC EXERCISE PROGRAMS AND EQUIPMENT

Isometric or static contraction is defined as a development of tension within a muscle without significant change in the length of its fibers. By this action, no motion or extra work is accomplished. In order to record tension developed in an isometric contraction, however, a slight shortening is allowed when maximal tension is desired, and the muscle is allowed to shorten as much as 10% of its original length.

Isometric Exercise Programs

Isometric exercise programs have the following effects and interactions:

• Isometric exercise programs can increase muscle strength and maintain these gains in muscle strengths.

• Maximal strength gains using isometric exercises may take up to eight weeks to develop.

• Muscular endurance is not increased with isometric training.

• Strength gains using an isometric program show a *position-dependent effect*. In other words, if a particular muscle group is trained isometrically at a specific joint angle, the muscle will show increased strength at that angle, but not necessarily at other angles.

- A muscle group that has been trained isometrically will show improved strength characteristics when this muscle is tested in a dynamic testing mode such as the Cybex II. These strength improvements are seen at low velocities but not at high velocities.

- Isometric exercise programs are effective in reducing atrophy of muscles that have been immobilized in plaster casts.

- Isometric exercise programs produce muscle hypertrophy.

- Proprioceptive neuromuscular facilitation increases maximal isometric contractions.

- Isometric contractions fatigue muscles rapidly. A fatiguing contraction is defined as a contraction greater than 15% of a maximum voluntary contraction.

- Full recovery of endurance following the fatiguing static contraction requires as long as 24 hours; 90% recovery occurs in the first hour.

- Fatiguing isometric contractions profoundly increase blood pressure (BP), heart rate, and cardiac output with little change in left ventricular stroke volume and no significant change in peripheral arterial vascular resistance (Table 1).

- The hypertensive response to isometric stress leads to a marked increase in left ventricular wall stress. The normal heart responds to this by maintaining a normal stroke volume and producing a slightly increased ventricular and diastolic pressure. The patient with mild congestive heart failure and decreased left ventricular function responds by showing a decreased stroke

TABLE 1.

Hemodynamic Responses to Exercise

Response	Isometric Increased...	Dynamic Increased...
Heart rate	Minimally	Markedly
Systolic BP	Markedly	Moderately
Diastolic BP	Markedly	. . .*
Mean BP	Markedly	. . .*
Cardiac output	Moderately	Markedly
Stroke volume	. . .*	Markedly
Systemic vascular pressure	. . .†	. . .†

*Decreased slightly.
†Unknown/unproven.

volume and an increase in diastolic pressure and a pressor response that increases the peripheral vascular resistance.

Equipment

To identify commercially available equipment designed for isometric exercise training, we obtained information from the following sources:

• The National Rehabilitation Information Center.

• ABLEDATA Custom Search Computer Program (accessed).

• Lumex Health Services, a subsidiary of Lumex, Inc., which produces Cybex and Eagle exercise equipment.

• The University of Vermont, Department of Physical Therapy.

• A local fitness store, i.e., a local franchise.

The results of these modes of search resulted in the identification of commercially available exercise equipment that is used solely for isometric exercise programs. The equipment identified was (1) a ergonomics isometric strength-testing unit, (2) a hand dynamometer, (3) listings of many isokinetics pieces of equipment that can also be used for isometric testings. (An example is the Cybex II when used at zero degree of rotation.)

From this search, there seems to be a scarcity or nonexistence of commercially available exercise equipment that is solely designed for isometric exercise programs. I believe that this is due to the fact that almost any heavy object or fixed structure can be used to do isometrics, such as a heavy chair, the arms of a chair, a wall, a piece of rope, and so forth. The scientific evidence to support the use of these structures is based on the scientific data presented about the efficacy of the isometric training programs.

Indications and Contraindications

The indications for use of isometric exercise programs are *to increase or preserve muscle strength and reduce muscle atrophy without moving the associated joint.* An example of this would be a patient with a fractured tibia in a long leg cast doing quadriceps exercises. Other indications are for patient convenience and the advantage of not needing sophisticated exercise equipment.

There are no contraindications to using an isometric exercise program when an exercise program is indicated, other than the drawbacks of the isometric program itself as compared with isotonic or isokinetic exercise programs. One relative contraindication is a patient with cardiovascular disease. Data show more stress on the cardiovascular system when the patient participates in isometric exercise programs than when the patient participates in isotonic programs.

Consensual Validation

The consensus of the panel on isometric equipment was:

GRIMSBY COLLEGE

LIBRARY

NUNS CORNER, GRIMSBY

- Isometric exercise will increase muscle strength and maintain strength gains.

- Muscular endurance is not increased by isometric training.

- Isometrically induced strength gains are position-dependent.

- Isometric exercise will produce muscle hypertrophy.

- There is a scarcity of commercially available exercise equipment designed solely for isometric exercise.

ISOMETRIC EXERCISE PROGRAMS AND EQUIPMENT RECOMMENDATIONS FOR FURTHER RESEARCH

We recommend scientific studies be conducted:

- To determine the frequency, duration, and specific joint angles at which exercise is necessary to maintain strength once an injured limb has reached a plateau in strength rehabilitation.

- To investigate the effect of isometric exercise on functional testing (i.e., the effect of isometric strength training on vertical leap).

ISOTONIC EXERCISE

Isotonic exercises are classically defined as meaning "constant tension." However, correct execution of free-weight exercises does not necessarily result in equal tension exerted by the muscle through its range of motion. Newton's second law states that the sum of all forces acting in a given direction equals the weight of the object being moved plus the mass and acceleration of that object. That is, the force generated by a muscle will be proportional to the acceleration of the weight through a range of motion. Each muscle group has its own individual strength curve based on the joint it is moving, its attachment sites, and limb length. This means that throughout the full range of motion for that particular joint and muscle group there will be both weak and strong points in the range of motion. The lifter will be able to exert only that amount of force which he is able to lift through the weakest point of the muscle curve. Because of the variable speed of constant resistance exercise, muscle development has proven unpredictable. Growing out of this inadequacy of isotonic exercise has been the development of variable exercise programs. Variable resistance exercise machines have been designed to accommodate individual strength curves for various muscle groups. Resistance is varied by the use of specially designed cams or various size pulleys all designed to vary the resistance to accommodate strength curves of a muscle group. The shape of these cams in placement of the pulleys has been empirical more than scientific. Designing an exercise machine for all individuals to match strength curves for one muscle group is at best difficult; and designing a machine to match strength curves for more than one muscle group or joint is practically impossible.

Isotonic exercise is referred to as either a positive exercise, i.e., concentric muscle contraction, or negative, i.e., eccentric muscle contraction. A concentric muscle contraction occurs when the muscle shortens as it resists a weight; an eccentric muscle contraction occurs if the muscle is lengthening as it performs work. Muscle can function "more efficiently" while eccentrically contracting than while concentrically contracting. That is, the muscle generates equal force with less resistance in the eccentric mode. Research has shown that the muscle develops selectively whether it is loaded eccentrically or concentrically. Eccentric strength gains are limited when only concentric modes are used; training with one mode fails to affect substantially the other. A recent trend toward development of isotonic exercise machines and exercise programs to include eccentric loading has occurred. The advantage of eccentric loading appears to be in development of muscle tension with less workload, which is particularly valuable when treating muscle tendon unit problems. The disadvantage of eccentric exercise is that there is documented increase muscle soreness as well as a need for specially designed equipment or the use of a weight-lifting partner to help perform this type of exercise. The amount of strength gained due to eccentric versus concentric or isotonic training may be greatly dependent on the proportion of resistance used for each type of training. What seems important is that any isotonic training program should include both forms of muscle contraction.

Isotonic Exercise Programs

All of the popular isotonic training regimens have one characteristic in common, namely, they employ a voluntary maximal contraction at some point during the training regimen. This concept was first introduced to the orthopedic literature in 1945 by DeLorme. DeLorme emphasized at that time the necessity of performing high-resistance exercises with a low number of repetitions. This was in contrast to exercise up to that time, which included multiple repetitions with low resistance. DeLorme accurately demonstrated rapid increases in muscle strength and bulk with high-resistance exercise.

DeLorme introduced the concept of progressive resistive exercises so that heavy weights would not be overemphasized and thereby injure the lifter. DeLorme's program consisted of one maximum voluntary contraction per week. There were no more than 15 "reps" per series with seven to ten series per exercise regimen. The lifter would then be tested at the end of each week to determine his maximum lifting capacity over ten repetitions. This would then establish the increase in weight for the following week. Using this approach, investigators have shown increases of over 5 lb in lean body weight with decreases in 5 lb of body fat in approximately eight weeks.

TABLE 2A.

The DAPRE Technique

Set	Portion of Working Weight Used	No. of Repetitions
1	1/2	10
2	3/4	6
3	Full	Maximum
4	Adjusted	Maximum

Because of the difficulty in establishing proper advancement schedules, Knight (1985) established the Daily Adjustable Progressive Resistive Exercise Program. The DAPRE program is designed to increase the amount of weight lifted over four series of repetitions (Tables 2A and 2B).

Another exercise regimen, i.e., the Oxford regimen, actually reverses this exercise scheme. In this regimen, the maximum amount of weight is lifted in the first series of repetitions and thereafter the weight is decreased over three series of ten repetitions. Comparing the various programs, investigators have failed to find any significant difference in increases in muscle strength and girth. One definite enhancement of these exercise routines was shown by Dickinson and Bennett (1985) where the use of high-repetition low-resistance exercises just before initiating high-resistance exercises yields significantly greater strength gains.

Studies comparing various types of training regimens are rare. Several researchers have made comparisons of strength gains by isokinetically and isotonically trained groups. All studies thus far have concluded that isokinetic training increases strength to a greater extent than isotonic training. Comparisons of isokinetic and isotonic contractions (by using electromyography) show that isokinetic contractions produce stronger and more consistent muscle contractions than isotonic exercises. Isokinetic training increases isokinetic strength and increases isotonic strength more than does training itself. This is especially true if isokinetic training is performed

TABLE 2B.

Guidelines for Adjustment of Working Weight

No. of Repetitions Performed During Set	Fourth Set	Adjustment to Working Weight Next Day
0–2	< 5–10 lb	Perform set over
3–4	< 5–10 lb	Keep the same
5–7	Keep the same	Up 5–10 lb
8–12	Up 5–10 lb	Up 5–15 lb
13 to . . .	Up 10–15 lb	Up 10–20 lb

at the faster velocities. When comparing isotonic to isometric exercise regimens, definite advantage to the isotonic exercise is seen. This of course depends on how individuals are tested. If isometric testing procedures are used, isometric training is superior to isotonic training. However, if dynamic testing procedures are used, isotonic training is superior to isometric in strength gains. Motor performance is improved to a greater extent by isotonic training than it is improved by isometric training. Increase in strength due to constant isotonic vs. variable resistance training appears controversial. Only one study demonstrates that variable resistance is superior to constant isotonic training.

Of particular caution when performing isotonic exercises is the "overwork syndrome." First delineated by Knowlton and Bennett (1957), it appears as though there is inability of the overworked muscle to sustain consistent contractions. The physiologic basis for this phenomenon has been undetermined, however. Many months are necessary for the muscle to recover properly and then properly respond to progressive resistive exercise.

Isotonic Equipment

A multitude of isotonic machines have come on the market in the last decade. Many of the machines serve a common purpose, i.e., strength gains through isotonic exercises. Some machines, i.e., Universal and N K products, allow both a concentric and eccentric exercise in the same repetition. Others, however, are termed "double-concentric" in that they exercise two different muscle groups in the same repetition, i.e., Merac. Despite the large number of commercially available exercise machines there seems to be only three major areas of change in the isotonic exercise area. First, machines were designed to vary the resistance and thereby accommodate individual muscle group strength curves. The second major change has been to isolate muscle and joint functions to individual exercise machines. Finally, the third major change has been to combine isotonic exercise with other modes, i.e., isometric and isokinetic exercise, through the use of robotic exercise machines.

Table 3 divides isotonic exercise machines into five subcategories and gives common examples of each. Advantages as well as disadvantages exist for each of these isotonic exercise types.

Free Weights.—The advantage of free weights has been, in the long-term experience, that they are available. Many scientific articles have confirmed the value of free weights in increasing lean body weight and reducing body fat. Free weights are inexpensive, convenient, and available to most people in need of strength training or rehabilitation. A major advantage that continues to maintain free weights as an important part of any isotonic exercise program is the ability to perform P and F exercises with them. Many weight lifters realize the value of free weights used through functional patterns. Disadvantages of free weight use include the potential for injury because of overload, the loading imbalance that exists with individual muscle strength curves, difficulty in isolating muscle groups (if this is desired) and the inability to control range of motion of the joint easily.

Weight Tables and Benches.—Combining free weights with weight stations, which include tables and benches, allows a more controlled motion during the exercise. This also enables better muscle group isolation and reduces the need for assistance during exercise. The dis-

TABLE 3.

Isotonic Exercise

Exercise Machine	Example
Free weights	Olympic
Weight tables & benches	N K products
Weight stations	Universal
Variable-resistance machines	Nautilus, Eagle
Robotic-assisted devices	Merac, KinCon

advantage of these exercise devices is that there is a limited ability to limit joint motion during exercise; also, the isotonic loading imbalance through the muscle strength curve still exists.

Weight Stations.—Starting in the 1960s, individual exercise machines were designed to isolate muscle and joint exercise. Introduced with this type of machine was circuit weight taining. Scientific articles comparing circuit weight training vs. free weights have been published that show evidence of superior cardiovascular enhancement with circuit weight training. No significant differences were demonstrated when muscle strength, girth, and lean body weight were measured. Other advantages of weight stations include adjustments to accommodate for different size weight lifters, better muscle isolation techniques, and better participant compliance based on ease of performance. The disadvantages with this type of weight training is that there continues to be a poor muscle force curve match with continued inability or difficulty in limiting joint motion with an inability to control joint speed.

Variable Resistance Machines.—The advantage of variable resistance machines has been alluded to previously. These devices attempt to match the resistance by the muscle with its individual strength curve. This allows more control loading with continued ability to isolate muscle function. These machines allow better posture adjustments as well as range of motion limiting capabilities. The disadvantages with these exercise devices is their cost, space requirements, and inability to control speed of exercise. There is serious doubt about their efficacy in accommodating muscle strength curves.

Robotic Machines.—More recently in the exercise machine market has been the advent of robotic exercise machines. These machines employ computer-controlled motor-driven resistance arms that not only resist movement but also can apply a force against the extremity being exercised. Because of the computer-enhanced capabilities of these devices there is a more individualized approach to the rehabilitation program, which combines isometric, isokinetic, and isotonic exercises. Range of motion control, speed control, and accurate resistance determination are all superior with exercise machines. These machines allow concentric and eccentric exercises to be performed in one repetition, in contrast to the double-concentric isokinetic machines. The major disadvantage to these devices is lack of experience and scientific documentation of proven efficacy. Because of the sophistication of these devices there is need for user education as well as operator sophistication. Mechanical breakdown is more apt to occur when compared with other isotonic exercise devices and because of their expense there is limited access to the general public.

Isotonic Exercise: Indications and Contraindications

Indications.—Perhaps the single most common indication for isotonic exercise has been the strengthening of normal muscle groups. The use of isotonic exercise and free weights has remained the sine qua non of body builders for many years. Just as important an indication is the rehabilitation of atrophied or weakened muscles secondary to injury or surgery. The type of exercise regimen should be varied to avoid the overload syndrome when rehabilitating atrophied or weakened muscles. Another important indication for isotonic exercise is the restoration of normal joint motion. Although gains in passive joint motion can be obtained through passive stretching, joint motion will only be maintained if muscle strength is gained simultaneously. Another important indication for isotonic exercise is neuromuscular facilitation, particularly after neurologic injury where restoration of muscle strength and coordination occur slowly.

Contraindications.—The contraindications to isotonic exercise are for the most part associated with disease processes about the musculotendinous unit or joint that it is acting upon. Joint arthrosis can be irritated secondary to compressive forces from isotonic exercise and may have to be decreased or avoided entirely. Joint swelling or inflammation also are contraindications to heavy resistive exercises. Because of the spinal reflex mechanism associated with joint swelling and inflammation, progressive resistive exercises fail to produce significant strength gains in this situation. A relative contraindication is joint instability. Isotonic exercise through a complete range of joint motion in this situation may aggravate joint laxity and lead to increasing symptoms of pain and crepitation. In this situation limitation of joint motion during exercise may be important. Early muscle exercise after neuromuscular injury can prolong neuromuscular recovery. Before instituting progressive resistive exercises, sufficient time must be allowed for nerve muscle or tendon healing to occur. Other types of exercise modes such as isometric should be employed in this situation.

Consensual Validation

- Muscles function more efficiently while eccentrically contracting than while concentrically contracting.

- Isokinetic training increases strength to a greater extent than isotonic training.

- Isotonic exercise is more effective in increasing strength than isometric exercise. Isotonic exercise helps to restore and maintain joint motion.

ISOTONIC EXERCISE: RECOMMENDATIONS FOR FURTHER RESEARCH

We recommend that scientific studies be conducted:

- To compare strength increases with constant vs. variable resistant training.

- To determine the effect of isotonic training on functional testing (i.e., the vertical leap).

- To document the efficacy of one type of isotonic exercise equipment compared to another (i.e., three-way vs. weight stations).

ISOKINETIC TRAINING

Isokinetic exercise is resistance exercise performed at a constant preset speed. The speed is kept constant by resistance accommodating to muscle effort (torque). As muscle effort increases, resistance increases maintaining the preset speed. The major theoretical advantage of isokinetic exercise is allowing maximal muscle tension through a full range of motion. This is not always possible with other forms of training.

The advantages of isokinetic vs. isotonic or isometric training are controversial, and these differences should be considered when designing testing, training, or rehabilitation programs. The advantages vary with the level of training, testing, or rehabilitation involved. Fortunately, numerous investigators have studied the accuracy and reliability of isokinetic equipment. The results are generally favorable.

An extensive database is now available that allows meaningful comparison studies. However, since isokinetic exercise is a relatively new technique and is rapidly changing, a thorough investigation into the indications, contraindications, and techniques for use should be conducted.

Advantages of Isokinetic Exercise

- Isokinetic exercise programs can develop strength efficiently in various muscle groups in normal individuals in a training mode.

- Isokinetic equipment can document and reproduce a performance test.

- Isokinetic equipment allows exercise throughout a velocity spectrum.

- Strength gains achieved in high speed training carry over to slower speeds.

- Isokinetics can produce moderate improvements in aerobic conditioning if used in a circuit-training format. However, isokinetics do not produce the same level of gain as other standard forms of aerobic conditioning such as running or swimming performed for the same length of time and degree of effort.

- High-speed isokinetic training can reduce fatigability.

- Improvement in quickness may be possible with isokinetic training if the training speeds match or surpass functional speeds.

Indications for Isokinetic Exercise

Testing.—The primary use of isokinetic equipment today that has scientific support is testing, which has three commonly used modes:

- Strength. Maximum force generated by muscle contraction through a range of motion.

- Power. Force moved through a range of motion in fixed time (usually tested at greater than 180 degrees per second).

- Endurance. Duration of repetitive exercise until peak force decreases 50%.

Training.—

- Strength

- Power

- Endurance

- Motor performance

- Aerobic conditioning if used in a circuit-training format.

Rehabilitation.—Most of the information on isokinetic rehabilitation is about knee rehabilitation. Data are also available on ankle and shoulder.

After injury or operation about the knee, the physician and therapist know that, during this period, muscle, tendon, bone ligament, and hyaline cartilage undergo disuse changes. Precisely when these structures return to normal has not been determined. The hyaline cartilage surface of a joint can be damaged if the sheer and compressive stresses of isokinetic training are applied before those surfaces return to normal.

Disadvantages of Isokinetic Exercise

- Isokinetic equipment machines cannot protect the user from him- or herself. The individual must know his or her own limitation and must understand the potential for injury. Since resistance accommodates to effort, an overly aggressive individual can do harm.

- Isokinetic equipment requires an on-sight calibration system, including weight and time checks. Computer or factory calibration thus far is unsatisfactory.

- Trained personnel are needed to collect and interpret data correctly.

- True eccentric training is not possible in the isokinetic mode.

- Several sources of potential dynamometer error

exist, including gravity effects of the limb, time of acceleration to preset speed, and recording of work performed at speeds below preset speed.

- Some isokinetic programs are not compatible with endurance training.

- Systolic BP, diastolic BP, and pressure-heart rate increase significantly with isokinetic exercise. The increase of the BP-heart rate product correlates with the degree of effort exerted.

Contraindications to Isokinetic Exercise

- Inadequate supervision during testing, training, or rehabilitation.

- Inadequate patient understanding of the isokinetic concept.

- Significant patellofemoral disease.

- Conditions in which anterior translation of the tibia could be detrimental to the knee joint (anterior cruciate ligament reconstruction).

- Soft-tissue swelling of an extremity or joint effusion.

- Thromboembolic disease.

- Cardiovascular disease.

- Abnormal hyaline cartilage secondary to disuse, immobilization or injury.

(Note: Isokinetic equipment manufacturers were contacted and invited to present scientific data before the committee. Only two companies responded and expressed interest.)

Cybex

Cybex has had several years of experience with iso-kinetic devices and has accumulated extensive data in the areas of testing and exercise training. Energy is not stored in the Cybex system. The system is entirely passive. It does not function as an active robotic device. It does not provide an eccentric mode of training or testing. The potential for catastrophic failure is minimal in this system.

The device can be set for isometric contraction at any point in the range of motion of a joint. Multiple joint capability is possible through various attachments to the main system. Visual feedback is provided by a dial or monitor. However, there is no mechanism to limit force provided by the user. The range of motion may be limited by mechanical stops attached to the goniometer. A torque bar attachment (antishear device) has been designed for the purpose of limiting anterior translation of the tibia with anterior cruciate ligament insufficiency or after anterior cruciate surgery. This device should be used with caution.

Kin-Com

This system provides isokinetic, isometric, and eccentric training potential. The eccentric mode requires the use of an active robotic system. This is controlled by a computer. The potential for catastrophic failure is present. Although no data are available documenting such occurrences, the safety features are of concern.

Consensual Validation

It was the consensus of the panel on isokinetic exercise that:

- Isokinetic exercise can efficiently develop strength in a normal individual in a training mode.

- Isokinetic equipment allows for exercise throughout a velocity spectrum.

- Strength gains achieved at high-speed isokinetic training carry over to slower speeds.

- Improvement in quickness may be possible only if isokinetic training occurs at speeds that match or surpass the functional speeds.

- Isokinetic equipment can document and reproduce the performance test.

ISOKINETIC TRAINING: RECOMMENDATIONS FOR RESEARCH

We recommend that scientific studies be conducted:

- To determine when it is safe to begin isokinetic exercise for the muscles surrounding an injured joint.

- To compare isokinetic rehabilitation using isokinetic exercise vs. isotonic exercise and the effect on functional performance.

- To compare joint stability following repair or reconstruction of acute ligament injuries rehabilitated in the isokinetic vs. isotonic exercise modality.

5 | Other Modalities: Continuous Passive Motion (CPM) Stationary Bicycle

Lyle Micheli, M.D.

Dale Daniel, M.D.

Richard Steadman, M.D.

CONTINUOUS PASSIVE MOTION

Continuous passive motion (CPM) is a technique of rehabilitation that involves, in simplest form, passive motion of an extremity through an externally applied force. There are at least 13 devices now being used to perform this function. These were first introduced clinically in Canada in 1978 and in the United States in 1982. The clinical use of CPM is based on the work of Dr. Robert Salter, which began in 1970. Based on animal work, primarily with rabbits, Salter demonstrated an enhanced rate of healing of articular cartilage and prevention of localized cartilage degeneration, degenerative arthritis, and intraarticular adhesion and effusion.

Subsequent clinical studies by Dr. Salter and others, including Dr. Herb Cruz, have shown a decreased incidence of deep pain thrombosis, decreased postoperative swelling, and significant decrease in postoperative medication used. Early joint motion has been shown to decrease intraarticular effusion.

The mechanisms by which CPM accomplishes these objectives are unknown. They may include direct cellular response to extensive stress or a general enhanced circulation. Continuous passive motion has been recommended for the early mobilization of infected joints, postoperative synovectomy, knee fractures, ligamentous repair, total knee joint replacement, or any incipient joint contracture.

Clinical Use and Indications

Continuous passive motion is used postoperatively to help relieve the patient's pain, improve the general circulation of the extremity, enhance the nutrition of the joint (in particular the articular cartilage), and prevent contractions and adhesions. At the present, clinical indications for CPM include postoperative rehabilitation and management following ligament repair or other intraarticular surgery, internal fixation of fractures (particularly articular fractures), synovectomy, joint manipulation for contracture, operations on the extremities or joints for infection, and total joint replacement. There are continuous passive motion devices available for both the upper and lower extremity. Primarily the units are used for the elbow and knee mobilization, although there are certain devices that can also be used to mobilize the ankle and shoulder.

Contraindications

There are few contraindications for the use of this device. The relative contraindication most evident would be a noncompliant patient or clinical situation in which lack of information or experience by nursing personnel or therapists would render the use of the device a risk to the patient.

Risks

The risks of the use of continued passive motion devices include disruption of the surgical repair or fracture fixation, hemorrhage in the immediate postoperative period, and malfunction of the device.

Rationale for Passive Motion Programs

The effect of stress deprivation on the connective tissue has been documented in numerous animal studies. The consistent feature of the gross appearance of the periarticular and synovial tissues of immobilized joints is fibrofatty connector tissue proliferation within the joint space. In a rat model, there was significant growth within 30 days of fibrofatty tissue over the cartilage and destruction of the cartilage in 60 days. Ulceration develops at cartilage contact points, with rate and severity depending on the rigidity of the mobilization and the degree of joint compression. There are secondary changes in the subchondral bone.

The biomechanical and biochemical response to stress alteration has been studied by Akeson and colleagues (1973) in San Diego in both the dog and rabbit models. Cast and internal fixation have been used to immobilize the hind limb. Biomechanical changes of the knee composite are evaluated with an apparatus called an arthrograph. Joint stiffness in the knee is measured in terms of a torque-angular deformation diagram. Following immobilization of two weeks, joint stiffness is seen as an increase in torque needed to move the joint and an increase in areas of hysteresis. A progressive stiffness was seen between the second and 12th week during the study.

Biomechanical changes in ligaments were noted with testing of the isolated-MCL-bone complex following nine weeks of immobilization. Load to failure under tension revealed a decrease in linear slope, ultimate load to failure, and energy absorbed to about one third of the control limb. The point of failure change from a mid-substance ligament tear seen in controls to an avulsion at the tibial attachment site. Animals that were mobilized after nine weeks of immobilization with cage activity for 12 weeks were studied. The medial collateral ligament recovery was near normal; however, the attachment site at the tibia remained weak and failure occurred at two thirds of the load compared with the control limb.

Numerous animal studies verify the point that stress deprivation results in rapid change in joint mechanics, while exercise results in a slow increase in strength of the connective tissues.

Other studies have evaluated the biochemical effects of immobilization. The water content of the connective tissue, which is normally 65 to 75%, decreases. It is believed the water serves as a spacer between individual collagen fibers, permitting discrete movement of one fiber past another. The largest change in stress-deprived tissues is a drop in the glycosaminoglycan (GAG) content, which reduces normal connective tissue pliability. The normal turnover of GAG is short, with a half-life in terms of days, as opposed to collagen, which has a turnover in terms of months to one to two years. It is believed that in the immobilized limb, there is a decrease in the rate of GAG production. A loss of GAG and water results in a decrease in fiber distance and friction with motion between fibers. Studies of collagen metabolism reveal collagen turnover continues at a reduced level. It is believed that randomly oriented fibers are produced, which result in cross-linking between preexisting fibers.

Beneficial Effects of Motion

Animal studies have revealed there is an increased clearance rate from the synovial joint with joint motion. Hemarthrosis is cleared more rapidly, large particles injected into the joint are cleared more rapidly. Septic joints recover with less cartilage destruction (Salter). Cartilage lesions have improved the healing rate (Salter). There is improved healing of sutured tendons, as shown in patellar tendon laceration of a rabbit model

(Salter). Gelberman et al. (1980), using a canine paw model, demonstrated that five minutes of passive motion two times daily markedly improved the healing of the suture flexor tendon. The healing of the moved tendon was more intrinsic, as opposed to the extrinsic healing of the completely immobilized paw. The tensile strength of the healed tendon was greater in the joint that was moved rather than immobilized. Inoue et al. (1978) reported improved healing in a dog model of the medial collateral ligament in the mobilized animal as opposed to the immobilized animal.

In conclusion, there is a wealth of laboratory literature to support the thesis that motion and stress are important to the maintenance of normal connective tissue and the healing of connective tissue. There is also literature to support that ion enhances blood flow, decreases pain, and may be a factor in neuromuscular retraining programs.

CONTINUOUS PASSIVE MOTION: RECOMMENDATIONS FOR FURTHER RESEARCH

We recommend that scientific research be conducted:

- To refine the dose-response curve and standardize protocols for its use. Much of this research could be done on animal models. It would lend itself to clinical controlled studies in humans.

- To differentiate protocols between the various clinical conditions indicated for use, such as after ligament repair, joint infection, or joint replacement.

- To develop equipment that delivers the basic clinical requirements of passive motion at an efficient cost-effective level.

- To investigate the practice of combining neuromuscular stimulation and continuous passive motion. Presently, two of the CPM devices on the market incorporate additional neuromuscular stimulation, but the relative benefits of this practice have not been determined.

- To document with human clinical studies the extensive laboratory animal work done by Dr. Salter and colleagues.

- To determine the relative decrease in postoperative swelling.

- To determine the rate of wound healing and the effects on the synovial tissue and articular cartilage responses.

- To investigate particular risks from stress and motion at the biomechanical level.

STATIONARY BICYCLE

The stationary bicycle, or bicycle ergometer, is one of the most widely available devices in fitness and health clubs, physical therapy facilities, and gyms. Even the simplest of these devices usually has some measurement device for calculating work output, adjustable seat and handlebar heights, and variable speed of operation. The lowest possible setting is 25 W on most machines, with the typical training range from 70 to 110 W of work.

The earliest work on measuring and enhancing aerobic fitness—using the maximum oxygen uptake, the VO_2 max, as a measurement—was done by Strans on cycle ergometers.

While the apparatus has been supplemented by treadmill testing in many situations now, the stationary bicycle still is used in cardiac rehabilitation, in testing or training persons who cannot run, and, with modifications, in training and testing upper extremities.

The protocol used in cardiac rehabilitation utilizes pulse rate, which is a safe and consistent parameter. Training is usually done in the midrange between resting pulse and maximum pulse rate. This will result in equivalent work output of approximately 70% VO_2 max, which appears to be independent of patient weight, height, and other factors.

While enhanced aerobic fitness is not specific to the rehabilitation of the extremity injured patient, it still is an important consideration, particularly for the athlete.

In addition, we know that describing aerobic fitness as cardiovascular fitness is incorrect, since the adaptive changes are occurring in the skeletal muscle bed, with cardiac or pulmonary changes secondary.

Indications

The first indication for using the stationary bicycle is to maintain aerobic fitness following illness, injury, or surgery. The second indication is exercise for the well leg when the opposite extremity is immobilized. It has been shown that exercise in the well leg has beneficial effects for the immobilized leg also. The third indication is rehabilitation of the injured extremity itself, specifically to increase the range of motion, endurance, strength, and power.

Contraindications

The contraindications for the use of the stationary bicycle in rehabilitation include the patient with limited motion at the knee or hip who has severe pain associated with the use of the cycle, and patients with patellar femoral disease or arthritis. Another contraindication is patients who have associated injuries or illnesses that render the use of the cycle by them unsafe.

Clinical Applications

- Clinical indications include rehabilitation of a patient with an injured or painful knee following knee surgery or for knee overuse injuries.

- The cyclergometer or stationary cycle may have specific indications for rehabilitation of a patient after anterior cruciate ligament surgery because of the low levels of anterior shear associated with the use of the device.

- The stationary cycle may have particular value for a patient who cannot run or swim as aerobic rehabilitative techniques because they cannot take the impacting of running or cannot swim.

- The stationary cycle could also be useful following ankle injury or surgery.

- The stationary cycle may be useful following back injury or surgery. Care must be taken to adjust the cycle so that the patient suffers no pain while performing the cycling activity.

- Certain patients with rheumatoid arthritis, multiple sclerosis, excessive weakness, or cachexia cannot tolerate other aerobic and endurance training devices, but they can still be rehabilitated effectively using the stationary cycle.

Cycling Validation

One study that had importance for the aerobic use of the stationary bicycle was done by Costill et al. in 1977. The study demonstrated that use of stationary cycling enhanced restoration of muscle aerobic enzymes in the postoperative period.

With cruciate ligament injury, a study presented in the *American Journal of Sports Medicine* in 1985 by Henning et al. demonstrated the lack of deformation of the cruciate ligament during cycling. In this study, measurement devices were implanted in the anterior cruciate ligament (ACL) of patients with second-degree ACL sprains. These patients were tested while doing various activities. The amount of deformation caused by each activity was compared with deformation from an 80-lb Lachman test. Cycling produced 7% as much elongation as an 80-lb Lachman test.

This can be compared with a one-leg half-squat at 21%, and the use of a 20-lb weight boot from full extension to 22 flexion, which created an 87 to 121% elongation as compared with the 80-lb Lachman test.

The study by Henning et al. supports the use of cycling for rehabilitation in the anterior cruciate injured patient, or after cruciate repair.

McLeod and Blackburn published a study in 1980 on the biomechanics of knee rehabilitation with cycling. This study also provided information useful to the rehabilitation in a knee ligament–injured patient. They demonstrated that the quadriceps can be effectively rehabilitated with cycling while placing minimal stresses on the anterior cruciate ligament, joint capsule, and posterior structures of the knee. By modifying the seat position and pedal positions, they could further decrease these forces. Gastrocnemius is more active during pedaling with the ball of the foot and with the leg extended (by the higher seat). A ligament can be protected from stress if the hamstring activity is enhanced while the gastrocnemius is reduced.

In the study McLeod and Blackburn (1980) found that 102° of knee flexion was necessary for cycling. They suggested a starting rpm of 40 for ten minutes. The goal was to progress to an rpm level of 60 and a work duration of 60 minutes. When this level was reached, they suggested that sprints be added.

The study noted that seat height played a role in the degree of activity of the gastrocnemius, quadriceps, and load to the anterior cruciate ligament and meniscotibial ligaments. They also felt that toe pedaling would be more effective than heel pedaling in protection for the anterior cruciate ligament in capsule structures.

An additional study done by Ericson and Nisell, published in the *American Journal of Sports Medicine* in 1986, lends further support to cycling as a rehabilitation device, and refined the parameters for its use. Their study of six healthy persons resulted in several important observations.

First, the anterior pedal position creates less anterior shear force on the anterior cruciate ligament. They were able to identify a midposition on the cycle when the tibiofibular shear force was quite low.

They then compared the compressive and shear forces of cycling with other activities. The comparison revealed that cycling had only a 1.2 body-weight compression force as compared with 2 to 4 times for normal walking, 4 times for stair climbing, 3 to 7 times when rising from a normal chair, and 2 to 3 times body-weight compression force when lifting a 12-kg burden.

Compressive force was reduced by a decrease in workload or an increase in saddle weight.

The authors also observed that the vastus medialis and lateralis appeared to be the muscle groups most involved in cycling. These two muscle groups had 54 and 50% of the maximal isometric electromyographic (EMG) activity, whereas the central rectus femoris muscle activity was lower (12% maximum EMG). They postulated that this was because the rectus femoris is a two-joint muscle. Thus, it would be necessary to address the strength and endurance of the rectus femoris in later phases of rehabilitation.

The anterior tibial shear force increased significantly when the posterior foot position was used instead of the anterior foot position. They suggested that this most likely was due to the increased extension of the knee. The stress was decreased by the anterior foot position.

STATIONARY BICYCLE: RECOMMENDATIONS FOR FURTHER RESEARCH

We recommend that scientific research be conducted:

• To develop and evaluate different cycle designs. Possibilities include cycles that employ a different body position such as the semireclining or reclining position of the patient; cycles with variable crank lengths, including a shorter crank to accommodate patients with a limited range of motion; and cycles that have interchangeable pedals with handgrips to be used interchangeably for both upper and lower extremity rehabilitation.

- To determine how much strength is attainable in the injured extremity when the cycle is used as a rehabilitation device. While it is a commonly held belief that restoration of complete strength can be obtained using resistive weight training, the ability of the cycle to obtain similar levels of strength, endurance, power, and range of motion following injury have not been well documented.

- To study the specific mechanics of cycling, as they relate to the biomechanics of the uninjured as well as the injured extremity.

Bibliography

HEAT MODALITIES

Introduction

Academy of Physical Medicine and Rehabilitation: Syllabus: Medical Knowledge Program in Physical Medicine and Rehabilitation, 1986.

DeLisa JA: *Rehabilitation Medicine: Principles and Practices*. Philadelphia, JB Lippincott Co, 1988.

Licht SH: *Therapeutic Heat and Cold*. New Haven, E Licht Publisher, 1965 (ed 2); 1982 (ed 3).

Lehmann SF, Warren CG, Scham SM: Therapeutic heat and cold. *Clin Orthop* 1974; 99:207–245.

Michlovitz SL, Wolf SL: *Thermal Agents in Rehabilitation*. Philadelphia, FA Davis Co, 1986.

Prentice WE: *Therapeutic Modalities in Sports Medicine*. St Louis, CV Mosby Co, 1986.

Superficial Heat Modalities

Abramson DI, Burnett C, Bell Y, et al: Changes in blood flow, oxygen uptake and tissue temperature produced by therapeutic physical agents: I. Effect of ultrasound. *Am J Phys Med* 1960; 39:51–62.

Abramson DI, Bell Y, Rejal H, et al: Changes in blood flow, oxygen uptake and tissue temperature produced by therapeutic physical agents: II. Effects of short wave diathermy. *Am J Phys Med* 1960; 39:87–95.

Abramson DI, Mitchell RE, Tuck S, et al: Changes in blood flow oxygen uptake and tissue temperature produced by topical application of wet heat. *Arch Phys Med* 1961; 42:305–318.

Bouman HD: Physical medicine in the clinical aspects of local heat application. *Phys Ther Rev* 1950; 30:507–510.

Boyd IA, Eyzguirre C, Matthews PBC, et al: *The Role of the Gamma System in Movement and Posture*. New York, Association for the Aid of Crippled Children, 1964.

Crockford GW, Hellon RF: Vascular responses of human skin to infra-red radiation. *J Physiol* 1959; 149:424–432.

Dancik D, Degroot A: Galvanism in the treatment of ecchymosis. *Arch Phys Med* 1951; 32:593–597.

Erdman WJ III, Stoner EK: Comparative heating effects of moistaire and hydrocollator hot packs. *Arch Phys Med* 1956; 37:71–74.

Fischer E, Solomon S: Physiological responses to heat and cold, in Licht S (ed): *Therapeutic Heat and Cold*. New Haven, E Licht Publisher, 1965, chap 4, p 126.

Gersten JW, Wakim KG, Stow RW, et al: A comparative study of the heating of tissues by near and far infrared radiation. *Arch Phys Med* 1949; 30:691–699.

Grant AE: Cryokinetics in treatment of painful conditions of the musculoskeletal system. *Arch Phys Med Rehabil* 1964; 45:233–238.

Greenberg RS: The effects of hot packs and exercise on local blood flow. *Phys Ther* 1972; 52:272–278.

Hardy JD: Physiological responses to heat and cold. *Annu Rev Physiol* 1950; 12:119–144.

Harris R: Iontophoresis, in Licht S (ed): *Therapeutic Electricity and Ultraviolet Radiation*. New Haven, E Licht Publisher, 1959, chap 4, pp 146–168.

Herrick JF: Temperatures produced in tissue by ultrasound: An experimental study using various technics. *J Acoust Soc Am* 1953; 25:12–16.

Humphreys PW, Lind AR: The blood flow through active muscle of the forearm during sustained handgrip contraction. *J. Physiol* 1963; 166:120–135.

Hyman C, Winsor T: History of plethysmography. *J Cardiovasc Surg* 1961; 2:508–518.

Kottke FJ: Deterioration of the bedfast patient: Causes and effects. *Publ Health Rep* 1965; 80:437–447.

Kottke FJ: Effects of limitation of activity on the human body. *JAMA* 1966; 196:825–830.

Lehmann JF: Diathermy, in Krusen FH, Kottke FJ, Ellwood PM (eds): *Handbook of Physical Medicine and Rehabilitation*. Philadelphia, WB Saunders Co, 1971, chap 11, pp 273–345.

Lehmann JF: Ultrasound therapy, in Licht S (ed): *Therapeutic Heat*, ed 2. New Haven, E Licht Publisher, 1965.

Lehmann JF, Brunner GD, McMillan JA, et al: Comparative study of the efficiency of shortwave, microwave and ultrasonic diathermy in heating the hip joint. *Arch Phys Med* 1959; 4:510–512.

Lehmann JF, Brunner GD, McMillan JA, et al: A comparative evaluation of temperature distributions produced by microwaves at 2456 and 900 megacycles in geometrically complex specimens. *Arch Phys Med* 1962; 43:502–507.

Lehmann JF, Brunner GD, McMillan JA, et al: Temperature distributions as produced by microwaves in specimens under therapeutic conditions. *Ann Phys Med* 1963; 7:121–132.

Lehmann JF, Brunner GD, McMillan JA, et al: Modifications of heating patterns produced by microwaves at the frequencies of 2456 and 900 megacycles by physiologic factors in the human. *Arch Phys Med* 1964; 45:555–563.

Lehmann JF, deLateur BJ: Heat and cold in the treatment of arthritis, in Licht S (ed): *Arthritis and Physical Medicine*. New Haven, E Licht Publisher, 1969, pp 315–378.

Lehmann JF, deLateur BJ: Therapeutic heat, in Lehmann JF (ed): *Therapeutic Heat and Cold*, ed 3. Baltimore, Williams & Wilkins Co, 1982, pp 404–562.

Lehmann JF, deLateur BJ: Cryotherapy, in Lehmann JF (ed): *Therapeutic Heat and Cold*, ed 3. Baltimore, Williams & Wilkins Co, 1982, pp 563–602.

Lehmann JF, deLateur BJ, Silverman DR: Selective heating effects of ultrasound in human beings. *Arch Phys Med* 1966; 47:331–339.

Lehmann JF, deLateur BJ, Warren CG, et al: Heating of joint structure by ultrasound. *Arch Phys Med* 1968; 49:28–30.

Lehmann JF, Erickson DSJ, Martin GM, et al: Comparison of ultrasonic and microwave diathermy in physical treatment of periarthritis of shoulder. *Arch Phys Med* 1954; 35:627–634.

Lehmann JF, Fordyce WE, Rathbun LA, et al: Clinical evaluation of new approach in treatment of contractures associated with hip fracture after internal fixation. *Arch Phys Med* 1961; 42:95–100.

Lehmann JF, Guy AW, Johnston VC, et al: Comparison of relative heating patterns produced in tissues by exposure to microwave energy at frequencies of 2456 and 900 megacycles. *Arch Phys Med* 1962; 43:69–76.

Lehmann JF, Johnstone VC, McMillan JA, et al: Comparison of deep heating by microwaves at frequencies 2456 and 900 megacycles. *Arch Phys Med* 1965; 46:307–314.

Lehmann JF, McMillan JA, Brunner GD, et al: Comparative study of the efficiency of shortwave, microwave and ultrasonic diathermy in heating the hip joint. *Arch Phys Med* 1959; 40:510–512.

Lehmann JF, McMillan JA, Brunner GD, et al: Heating patterns produced in specimens by microwaves of the frequency of 2456 megacycles when applied with the "A, B, and C" directors. *Arch Phys Med* 1965; 46:307–314.

Lehmann JF, Silverman DR, Baum BA, et al: Temperature distribution in the human thigh produced by infrared, hot pack and microwave application. *Arch Phys Med* 1966; 47:291–299.

Lehmann JF, Stonebridge JB, deLateur BJ, et al: Temperatures in human thighs after hot pack treatment followed by ultrasound. *Arch Phys Med* 1978; 59:472–476.

Lehmann JF, Warren CG, Scham SM: Therapeutic heat and cold. *Clin Orthop* 1974; 99: 207–245.

Lehmkuhl D, Imig CJ: Measurement of maximal blood flow following standardized fatiguing exercise for evaluation of the functional capacity of the peripheral circulation. *Am J Phys Med* 1961; 40:146–157.

Lewis T, Love WS: Vascular reactions of the skin to injury: III. Some effects of freezing, of cooling and warming. *Heart* 1926; 13:27–60.

Licht S (ed): *Therapeutic Heat.* New Haven, E Licht Publisher, 1958.

Licht S (ed): *Therapeutic Exercise.* New Haven, E Licht Publisher, 1961.

Martin GM, Herrick JF: Further evaluation of heating by microwaves and by infrared as used clinically. *JAMA* 1955; 159:1286–1287.

Mead S, Knott M: Topical cryotherapy: Use for relief of pain and spasticity. *Calif Med* 1966; 105:179–181.

Morrison WF, Parrish JA, Fitzpatrick TE: Controlled study of PUVA and adjunctive topical therapy in the management of psoriasis. *Br J Dermatol* 1978; 98:125–132.

Morrissey LJ: Effects of pulsed short-wave diathermy upon volume blood flow through the calf of the leg. *Phys Ther* 1966; 46:946–952.

Schull JR: Heating modalities. *South Med J* 1968; 61:621–624.

Schwan HP: The biophysical basis of physical medicine. *JAMA* 1956; 160:191–197.

Schwan HP: Biophysics of diathermy, in Licht S (ed): *Therapeutic Heat.* New Haven, E Licht Publisher, 1958.

Schwan HP, Garstensen EL: Application of electric and acoustic impedance measuring techniques to problems in diathermy. *Trans Am Instr Elec Eng* 1953; 72:106.

Selke OO Jr: Histamine iontophoresis to prevent tissue necrosis following levarterenol extravasation. *Arch Phys Med* 1956; 37:643–646.

Stillwell GK: Therapeutic heat, in Krusen FH, Kottke

FJ, Elwood PM (eds): *Handbook of Physical Medicine and Rehabilitation*. Philadelphia, WB Saunders Co, 1971, chap 10, pp 273–345.

Sweeney FX, Horvath SM, Mellette HC, et al: Infrared heating of tissues. *Arch Phys Med* 1950; 31:493–501.

Sweeney FX, Stoner EK: Hot packing. *Arch Phys Med* 1951; 32:206–210.

Wells HS: Temperature equalization for the relief of pain: An experimental study of the relation of thermal gradients to pain. *Arch Phys Med* 1947; 28:135–139.

Diathermy: Shortwave and Microwave

Diagnostic and therapeutic technology assessment (DATTA): Diathermy (question and answer). *JAMA* 1983; 250:540.

Farrell JP, Twomey LT: Acute low back pain: Comparison of two conservative treatment approaches. *Med J Aust* 1982; 1:160–164.

Gibson T, Grahame R, Harkness J, et al: Controlled comparison of short-wave diathermy treatment with osteopathic treatment in nonspecific low back pain. *Lancet* 1985: 1(8440):1248–1261.

Guerquin-Kern JL, Palas L, Priou A, et al: Local hyperthermia using microwaves for therapeutic purpose: Experimental studies of various applicators. *J. Microwave Power* 1981; 161:305–311.

Hillman SK, Delforge G: The use of physical agents in rehabilitation of athletic injuries. *Clin Sports Med* 1985; 4:431–438.

Holfand AE, Bruno J: Therapeutic modalities and procedures: I. Cold and heat. *Clin Podiatry* 1984; 1:301–313.

Lau RWM, Dunscombe PB: Notes: Some observations on stray magnetic fields and power outputs from short-wave diathermy equipment. *Health Phys* 1984; 46:939–943.

Lehmann JF, McDougall JA, Guy AW, et al: Heating patterns produced by shortwave diathermy applicators in tissue substitute models. *Arch Phys Med Rehabil* 1983; 64:575–577.

Mosely H, Davison M: Exposure of physiotherapists to microwave radiation during microwave diathermy treatment. *Clin Phys Physiol Meas* 1981; 2:217–221.

Policoff LD: Effective use of physical modalities. *Orthop Clin North Am* 1982; 13:579–586.

Sekins M, Lehmann JF, Esselman P, et al: Local muscle blood flow and temperature responses to 915 mHz diathermy as simultaneously measured and numerically predicted. *Arch Phys Med Rehabil* 1984; 65:1–7.

Stuckly MA, Repacholi MH, Leeuyer DW, et al: Exposure to the operator and patient during short wave diathermy treatments. *Health Phys* 1982; 42:341–366.

Therapeutic Ultrasound

Binder A, Hodge G, Greenwood AM, et al: Is therapeutic ultrasound effective in treating soft tissue lesions? *Br Med J [Clin Res]* 1985; 290(6467):512–514.

Brust M, Toback S, Benton JG: Some effects of ultrasound and of temperature on the contractions of isolated mammalian skeletal muscle. *Arch Phys Med Rehabil* 1969; 50:677–694.

Currier DP, Greathouse D, Swift T: Sensory nerve conduction: Effect of ultrasound. *Arch Phys Med Rehabil* 1978; 59:181–185.

Delacerda FG: Ultrasonic techniques for treatment of plantar warts in athletes. *J Orthop Sports Phys Ther* 1979; 1:100–102.

Downing DS, Weinstein A: Ultrasound therapy of subacromial bursitis: A double blind trial. *Phys Ther* 1986; 66:194–199.

Dyson M, Pond JB: The effect of pulsed ultrasound on tissue regeneration. *Physiotherapy* 1970; 56:136–142.

Dyson M, Suckling J: Stimulation of tissue repair by ultrasound: A survey of mechanisms involved. *Physiotherapy* 1978; 64:105–108.

Farmer WC: Effect of intensity of ultrasound on conduction velocity of motor axons. *Phys Ther* 1968; 48:1233–1237.

Gersten JW: Effect of metallic objects on temperature rises produced in tissue by ultrasound. *Am J Phys Med* 1958; 37:75–82.

Gersten JW: Non-thermal neuromuscular effects of ultrasound. *Am J Phys Med* 1958; 37:235–236.

Griffin JE, Echternach JL, Price RE, et al: Patients treated with ultrasonic driven hydrocortisone and with ultrasound alone. *Phys Ther* 1967; 47:594–601.

Griffin JE, Karselis TC: *Physical Agents for Physical Therapists*, ed 2. Springfield, Ill, Charles C Thomas Publisher, 1982.

Griffin JE, Touchstone JC: Low-intensity phonophoresis of cortisol in swine. *Phys Ther* 1968; 48:1336–1344.

Griffin JE, Touchstone JC: Effects of ultrasonic frequency on phonophoresis of cortisol into swine tissues. *Am J Phys Med* 1972; 51:62–78.

Hashish I, Harvey W, Harris M: Anti-inflammatory effects of ultrasound therapy: Evidence for a major placebo effect. *Br J Rheumatol* 1986; 253:77–81.

Kleinkort JA, Wood F: Phonophoresis with one percent versus ten percent hydrocortisone. *Phys Ther* 1975; 55:1320–1324.

Klug W, Franke WG, Knoch HG: Scintigraphic control of bone-fracture healing under ultrasonic stimulation: An animal experimental study. *Eur J Nucl Med* 1986; 11:494–497.

Kramer JF: Effect of therapeutic ultrasound intensity on subcutaneous tissue temperature and ulnar nerve conduction velocity. *Am J Phys Med* 1985; 64:1–9.

Lehmann JF, deLateur BJ, Warren CG, et al: Heating of joint structures by ultrasound energy. *Arch Phys Med Rehabil* 1968; 49:28–30.

Lehmann JF, Masock AJ, Warren CG, et al: Effects of therapeutic temperatures on tendon extensibility. *Arch Phys Med Rehabil* 1970; 51:481–487.

Madsen PW, Gersten JW: The effect of ultrasound conduction velocity of peripheral nerve. *Arch Phys Med Rehabil* 1961; 42:645–649.

Michlovitz SL: *Thermal Agents in Rehabilitation*. Philadelphia, FA Davis Co, 1986.

Stevenson JH, Pang CY, Linsay WK, et al: Functional, mechanical, and biomechanical assessment of ultrasound therapy on tendon healing in the chicken toe. *Plast Reconstr Surg* 1986; 77:965–972.

Vaughn DT: Direct method versus underwater method in the treatment of plantar warts with ultrasound: A comparative study. *Phys Ther* 1973; 53:396–397.

Vaughn JL, Bender LF: Effects of ultrasound on growing bone. *Arch Phys Med Rehabil* 1959; 40:158–160.

Laser

Saperia D, Glassberg E, Lyons RF, et al: Demonstration of elevated type I and type III procollagen mRNA levels in cutaneous wounds treated with helium-neon laser. *Biochem Biophys Res Commun* 1986; 138:1123–1128.

Seitz LM, Kleinkort JA: Low-power laser: Its applications in physical therapy, in Michlovitz SL: *Thermal Agents in Rehabilitation*. Philadelphia, FA Davis Co, 1986.

COLD MODALITIES (CRYOTHERAPY)

Abramson DI, Chu LS, Tuck S Jr, et al: Effect of tissue temperatures and blood flow on motor nerve conduction velocity. *JAMA* 1966; 198:1082–1088.

Barnes L: Cryotherapy: Putting injury on ice. *Physician Sports Med* 1979; 3:130–136.

Brooks B, Duncan G: The influence of temperature on wounds. *Ann Surg* 1941; 114: 1069–1075.

Clarke R, Hellon R, Lind A: Vascular reactions of the human forearm to cold. *Clin Sci* 1958; 17:165–179.

Drez D, Faust DC, Evans JP: Cryotherapy and nerve palsy. *Am J Sports Med* 1981; 9:256–257.

Kalanak A, Medlar CE, Fleagle SB, et al: Athletic injuries: Heat vs. cold. *Am Fam Physician* 1975; 12:131–134.

Kellett J: Acute soft tissue injuries: A review of the literature. *Med Sci Sports Exerc* 1986; 18:489–500.

Knight KL: *Cryotherapy: Theory, Technique, and Physiology*. Chattanooga, Tenn, Chattanooga Corp, 1985.

Lehmann JF: *Therapeutic Heat and Cold*, ed 3. Baltimore, Williams & Wilkins Co, 1982.

Lewis T: Observations upon the reactions of vessels of the human skin to cold. *Heart* 1930; 15:177–208.

Lowdon BJ, Moore RJ: Determinants and nature of intramuscular temperature changes during cold therapy. *Am J Phys Med* 1975; 54:223–233.

Matsen FA III, Questad K, Matsen AL, et al: The effect of local cooling on postfracture swelling. *Clin Orthop* 1975; 109:201–205.

McMaster WC: A literary review on ice therapy in injuries. *Am J Sports Med* 1977; 5:124–126.

McMaster WC: Cryotherapy. *Physician Sports Med* 1982; 10:112–119.

McMaster WC, Liddle S: Cryotherapy: An influence on posttraumatic limb edema. *Clin Orthop* 1980; 150:283–287.

McMaster WC, Liddle S, Waugh TR: Laboratory evaluation of various cold therapy modalities. *Am J Sports Med* 1978; 6:291–294.

Meeusen R, Lievens P: The use of cryotherapy in sports injuries. *Sports Med* 1986; 3:398–414.

Rusk HA: *Rehabilitation Medicine*. St Louis, CV Mosby Co, 1977.

Waylonis GW: The physiological effects of ice massage. *Arch Phys Med Rehabil* 1967; 48:37–42.

Yackzaw L, Adams C, Francis KT: The effects of ice massage on delayed muscle soreness. *Am J Sports Med* 1984; 12:159–165.

ELECTRICAL STIMULATION

Andersson SA, Hansson G, Holmgren E, et al: Evaluation of the pain suppressive effect of different frequencies of peripheral electrical stimulation in chronic pain conditions. *Acta Orthop Scand* 1976; 47:149–157.

Arvidsson I, Arvidsson H, Eriksson E, et al: Prevention of quadriceps wasting after mobilization: An evaluation of the effect of electrical stimulation. *Orthopedics* 1986; 9:1519–1528.

Arvidsson I, Eriksson E: Postoperative TENS pain relief after knee surgery: Objective evluation. *Orthopedics* 1986; 9:1346–1351.

Bishop B: Pain: Its physiology and rationale for management. Part I. Neuroanatomical substrate of pain. *Phys Ther* 1980; 60(1):13–20.

Bodenheim R, Bennett JH: Reversal of a Sudeck's atrophy by the adjunctive use of transcutaneous electrical nerve stimulation: A case report. *Phys Ther* 1983; 63:1445–1447.

Boutelle D, Smith B, Malone T: A strength study utilizing the electro-stim 180. *J Orthop Sports Phys Ther* 1985; 7:50–53.

Cooperman AM, Hall B, Mikalacki K: Use of transcutaneous electrical stimulation in the control of postoperative pain. *Am J Surg* 1977; 133:185–187.

Cornell PE, Lopez AL, Malofsky H: Pain reduction with transcutaneous electrical nerve stimulation after foot surgery. *J Foot Surg* 1984; 23:326–333.

Currier DP, Lehmann J, Lightfoot P: Electrical stimulation of the quadriceps femoris muscle. *Phys Ther* 1979; 59:1508–1512.

Currier DP, Mann R: Muscular strength development by electrical stimulation in healthy individuals. *Phys Ther* 1983; 63:915–921.

Currier DP, Mann R: Pain complaint: Comparison of electrical stimulation with conventional isometric exercise. *J Orthop Sports Phys Ther* 1984; 5:318–323.

Dlin RA, Benmair A, Hanne N: Pain relief in sports injuries: Application of TENS to acupuncture points. *Int J Sports Med* 1980; 1:203–206.

Dwyer AF: The use of electrical current stimulation in spinal fusion. *Orthop Clin North Am* 1975; 6:265–272.

Eriksson E: Rehabilitation of muscle function after

sport injury: Major problem in sports medicine. *Int J Sports Med* 1981; 2:1–6.

Eriksson E, Haggmark T: Comparison of isometric muscle training and electrical stimulation supplementing isometric muscle training in the recovery after major knee ligament surgery: A preliminary report. *Am J Sports Med* 1979; 7:169–171.

Eriksson E, Haggmark T, Kiessling KH, et al: Effects of electrical stimulation on human skeletal muscle. *Int J Sports Med* 1981; 2:18–22.

Ersek RA: Low-back pain. Prompt relief with transcutaneous neuro-stimulation: A report of 35 consecutive patients. *Orthop Rev* 1976; 5:27–31.

Ersek RA: Transcutaneous electrical neurostimulation. *Clin Orthop* 1977; 128:314–324.

Frank C, Schachar N, Dittrich D, et al: Electromagnetic stimulation of ligament healing in rabbits. *Clin Orthop* 1983; 175:263–272.

Fried T, Johnson R, McCracken W: Transcutaneous electrical nerve stimulation: Its role in the control of pain. *Arch Phys Med Rehabil* 1984; 65:228–231.

Garhammer J: An introduction to the use of electrical muscle stimulation with athletes. *NSCA J* 1983; 5:44–45.

Gersh MR, Wolf SL, Rao VR: Evaluation of transcutaneous electrical nerve stimulation for pain relief in peripheral neuropathy: A clinic documentation. *Phys Ther* 1980; 60:48–52.

Gersh MR, Wolf SL: Applications of transcutaneous electric nerve stimulation in the management of patients with pain: State of the art update. *Phys Ther* 1985; 65:314–321.

Gould N, Donnermeyer D, Pope M, et al: Transcutaneous muscle stimulation to retard disuse atrophy after open meniscectomy. *Clin Orthop* 1983; 178:190–197.

Halbach JW, Straus D: Comparison of electromyostimulation to isokinetic training increasing power of the knee extensor mechanism. *J Orthop Sports Phys Ther* 1980; 2:20–24.

Harris WH, Moyen BJ-L, Thrasher EL, et al: Differential response to electrical stimulation: A distinction between induced osteogenesis intact tibiae and the effect on fresh fracture effects in radii. *Clin Orthop* 1977; 124:31–40.

Hartsell HS: Electrical muscle stimulation and isometric exercise effects on selected quadriceps parameters. *J Orthop Sports Phys Ther* 1986; 8:203–209.

Harvie KW: A major advance in control of postoperative knee pain. *Orthopedics* 1979; 2:26–27.

Hassler CR, Rybicki EF, Diegle RB, et al: Studies in enhanced bone healing via electrical stimuli: Comparative effectiveness of various parameters. *Clin Orthop* 1977; 124:9–19.

Hughes GS Jr, Lichstein PR, Whitlock D, et al: Response of plasma beta-endorphins to transcutaneous electrical nerve stimulation in healthy subjects. *Phys Ther* 1984; 64:1062–1066.

Jacobs JD, Norton LA: Electrical stimulation of experimental nonunions. *Clin Orthop* 1981; 161:146–153.

Jensen JE, Conn RR, Hazelrigg G, et al: The use of transcutaneous neural stimulation and isokinetic testing in arthroscopic knee surgery. *Am J Sports Med* 1985; 13:27–33.

Jimenez W, Griend RV: The use of TENS following hip replacement surgery. *Orthop Rev* 1985; 14:706–708.

Jorgensen TE: Electrical stimulation of human fracture healing by means of a slow pulsating, asymmetrical direct current. *Clin Orthop* 1977; 124:124–142.

Kane K, Taub A: A history of local electrical analgesia. *Pain* 1975; 1:124–138.

Kramer JF, Mendryk SW: Electrical stimulation as a strength improvement technique: A review. *J Orthop Sports Phys Ther* 1982; 4:91–98.

Kramer J, Linsay D, Magee D, et al: Comparison of voluntary and electrical stimulation contraction torques. *J Orthop Sports Phys Ther* 1984; 5:324–331.

Kubiak RJ Jr, Whitman KM, Johnston RM: Changes in quadriceps femoris muscle strength using isometric exercise versus electrical stimulation. *J Orthop Sports Phys Ther* 1987; 8:537–541.

Lampe GN: Introduction to the use of transcutaneous electrical nerve device. *Phys Ther* 1978; 58:1450–1454.

Laughman RK, Youdas JW, Garrett TR, et al: Strength changes in the normal quadriceps femoris muscle as a result of electrical stimulation. *Phys Ther* 1983; 63:494–499.

Lehmann TR, Russell DW, Spratt KF: The impact of patients with nonorganic physical findings on a controlled trial of transcutaneous electrical nerve stimulation and electroacupuncture. *Spine* 1983; 8:625–634.

Lewis D, Lewis B, Sturrock RD: Transcutaneous electrical nerve stimulation in osteoarthrosis: A therapeutic alternative? *Ann Rheum Dis* 1984; 43:47–49.

Melzack R: Prolonged relief of pain by brief, intense transcutaneous somatic stimulation. *Pain* 1974; 1:357–373.

Melzack R: *The Puzzle of Pain.* New York, Basic Books Inc, 1973.

Melzack R, Vetere P, Finch L: Transcutaneous electrical nerve stimulation for low back pain: A comparison of TENS and massage for pain and range of motion. *Phys Ther* 1983; 63:489–493.

Mohr T, Carlson B, Sulentic C: Comparison of isometric exercise and high volt galvanic stimulation on quadriceps femoris muscle strength. *Phys Ther* 1985; 65:606–612.

Morrissey MC, Brewster CE, Shields, et al: The effects of electrical stimulation on the quadriceps during postoperative knee immobilization. *Am J Sports Med* 1985: 13:40–45.

Nashold BS, Goldner JL, Mullen JB, et al: Long-term pain control by direct peripheral-nerve stimulation. *J Bone Joint Surg* 1982; 64A:1–10.

Nobbs LA, Rhodes EC: The effect of electrical stimulation and isokinetic exercise on muscular power of the quadriceps femoris. *J Orthop Sport Phys Ther* 1986; 8:260–268.

O'Brien WJ, Rutan FM, Sanborn C, et al: Effect of transcutaneous electrical nerve stimulation on human blood beta-endorphin levels. *Phys Ther* 1984; 64:1367–1374.

Olsen GA, Rosen H, Hohn RB: Electrical muscle stimulation as a means of correcting induced canine scoliotic curves. *Clin Orthop* 1977; 125:227–235.

Owens J, Malone T: Treatment parameters of high frequency electrical stimulation as established on the Electro-stim 180. *J Orthop Sports Phys Ther* 1983; 4:162–168.

Paterson DC, Carter RF, Tilbury RF, et al: The effects of varying current levels of electrical stimulation. *Clin Orthop* 1982; 169:303–312.

Paterson DC, Hillier TM, Carter RF, et al: Experimental delayed union of the dog tibia and its use in assessing the effect of an electrical bone growth stimulator. *Clin Orthop* 1977: 128:340–350.

Peckham PH, Mortimer JT, Marsolais EB: Alteration in the force and fatigability of skeletal muscles in quadriplegic humans following exercise induced by chronic electrical stimulation. *Clin Orthop* 1976; 114:326–334.

Prentice WE: *Therapeutic Modalities in Sports Medicine.* St Louis, CV Mosby Co, 1986.

Ray CD: Electrical stimulation: New methods for therapy and rehabilitation. *Scand J Rehabil Med* 1978; 10:65–74.

Roeser WM, Meeks LW, Venis R, et al: The use of transcutaneous nerve stimulation for pain control in athletic medicine: A preliminary report. *Am J Sports Med* 1976; 4:210–213.

Romano RL, Burgess EM, Rubenstein CPO: Percutaneous electrical stimulation for clinical tibial fracture repair. *Clin Orthop* 1976; 114:290–294.

Romero JA, Sanford TL, Schroeder RV, et al: The effects of electrical stimulation of normal quadriceps on strength and girth. *Med Sci Sports Exer* 1982; 14:194–197.

Rosenburg MR, Curtis L, Bourke DL: Transcutaneous electrical nerve stimulation for the relief of postoperative pain. *Pain* 1978; 5:129–133.

Selkowitz DM: Improvement in isometric strength of the quadriceps femoris muscle after training with electrical stimulation. *Phys Ther* 1985; 65:186–196.

Shenton DW Jr, Heppenstall RB, Chance B, et al: Electrical stimulation of human muscle studied using 31P-nuclear magnetic resonance spectroscopy. *J Orthop Res* 1986; 4:204–211.

Sheon RP: Transcutaneous electrical nerve stimulation from electric eels to electrodes. *Postgrad Med* 1984; 75:71–74.

Sjolund B, Eriksson E: Endorphins and analgesia produced by peripheral conditional stimulations. *Adv Pain Res Ther* 1979; 3:587–592.

Smith J, Romansky N, Vomero J, et al: The effect of electrical stimulation on wound healing in diabetic mice. *J Am Podiatr Med Assoc* 1984; 74:71–74.

Smith MJ: Electrical stimulation for relief of musculoskeletal pain. *Phys Sports Med* 1983; 11:47–55.

Smith MJ, Hutchins RC, Hehenberger D: Transcutaneous neural stimulation use in postoperative knee rehabilitation. *Am J Sports Med* 1983; 11:75–82.

Solomonow M, Shoji H, King A, et al: Studies toward spasticity suppression with high frequency electrical stimulation. *Orthopedics* 1984; 7:1284–1288.

Solomonow M, Baratta R, Miwa T, et al: A technique for recording the EMG of electrically stimulated skeletal muscle. *Orthopedics* 1985; 8:492–495.

Soric R, Devlin M: Transcutaneous electrical nerve stimulation: Practical aspects and applications. *Postgrad Med* 1985; 78(4):101–107.

Spadaro JA: Electrically stimulated bone growth in animal and man: Review of the literature. *Clin Orthop* 1977; 122:325–332.

Strivastava KP, Saxena AK: Electrical stimulation in delayed union of long bones. *Acta Orthop Scand* 1977; 48:562–565.

Strivastava KP, Lahiri V, Khare A, et al: Histomor-phologic evidence of fracture healing after direct electrical stimulation in dogs. *J Trauma* 1982; 22:785–786.

Standish WD, Valiant GA, Bonen A, et al: The effects of immobilization and of electrical stimulation on muscle glycogen and myofibrillar ATPase. *Can J Appl Sports Sci* 1982; 7:267–271.

Kane K, Taub A: A history of local electrical analgesia. *Pain* 1975; 1:125–138.

Tseng LF, Loh HH, Li CH: Beta endorphin as a potent analgesic by intravenous injection. *Nature* 1976; 263:239–240.

VanderArk GD, McGrath KA: Transcutaneous electrical stimulation in treatment of postoperative pain. *Am J Surg* 1975; 130:338–340.

Vodovnik L, Kralj A, Stanic U, et al: Recent applications of functional electrical stimulation to stroke patients in Ljubljana. *Clin Orthop* 1978: 131:64–70.

Wakim KG: A review of denervation atrophy with some comment on the results of electric stimulation in humans and in animals. *Clin Orthop* 1958; 12:63–73.

Walmsley RP, Letts G, Vooys J: A comparison of torque generated by knee extension with a maximal voluntary muscle contraction vis-a-vis electrical stimulation. *J Orthop Sports Phys Ther* 1984; 6:10–17.

Waters RL, McNeal D, Perry J: Experimental correction of footdrop by electrical stimulation of the peroneal nerve. *J Bone Joint Surg* 1975; 57A:1047–1054.

Williams RA, Morrissey MC, Brewster CE: The effect of electrical stimulation on quadriceps strength and thigh circumference in meniscectomy patients. *J Orthop Sports Phys Ther* 1986: 8:143–146.

Wolf SL: Perspectives on CNS responsiveness to TENS. *Phys Ther* 1978; 58:1443–1449.

THERAPEUTIC EXERCISE MODALITIES

Isometric Exercise

Bender JA, Kaplan HM: The multiple angle testing

method for the evaluation of muscle strength. *J Bone Joint Surg* 1963; 45A:135–140.

Edwards RH, Hill DK, Jones DA, et al: Fatigue of long duration in human skeletal muscle after exercise. *J Physiol (London)* 1977; 272:769–778.

Funderburk CF, Hipskind SG, Welton RF, et al: Development of and recovery from fatigue induced by static effort at various tensions. *J Appl Physiol* 1974; 37:392–396.

Gardner GW: Specificity of strength changes of the exercised and nonexercised limb following isometric training. *Res Q* 1963; 34:98–101.

Helfant RH, De Villa MA, Meister SG: Effect of sustained isometric and grip exercise on left ventricular performance. *Circulation* 1971; 44:982–993.

Hettinger T: *Physiology of Strength.* Springfield, Ill, Charles C Thomas Publisher, 1961, p 82.

Karpovich PV: *Physiology of Muscular Activity.* Philadelphia, WB Saunders Co, 1959.

Kivowitz C, Parley WW, Donosco R, et al: Effects of isometric exercise on cardiac performance: The grip test. *Circulation* 1971: 14:994–1002.

Lind AR: Muscle fatigue and recovery from fatigue induced by sustained contractions. *J. Physiol (London)* 1959: 147:162–171.

Lind M: Increase of muscle strength from isometric quadriceps exercises at different knee angles. *Scand J Rehabil Med* 1979; 22:33–36.

MacConaill MA, Basmajian JV: *Muscles and Movements: A Basis for Human Kinesiology.* Baltimore, Williams & Wilkins Co, 1969, p 421.

McMorris RO, Elkins EC: A study of production and evaluation of muscular hypertrophy. *Arch Phys Med* 1954; 35:420–426.

Merton PA: Voluntary strength and fatigue. *J Physiol (London)* 1954; 123:553–564.

Moore JC: Active resistive stretch and isometric exercise in strengthening wrist flexion in normal adults. *Arch Phys Med Rehabil* 1971; 52:264.

Muller EA: Training muscle strength. *Ergonomics* 1959; 2:216–222.

Muller EA: Physiology of muscle training. *Rev Can Biol* 1962; 21:303–313.

Quinones MA, Gaasch WH, Waisser E, et al: An analysis of left ventricular response to isometric exercise. *Am Heart J* 1974; 88:29–36.

Rasch PJ, Morehouse LE: Effect of static and dynamic exercises on muscle strength and hypertrophy. *J Appl Physiol* 1957; 11:29–34.

Rohmert W: Untersuchung statischer Haltearbeiten in achtstundigen Arbeitsversuchen. *Int Z Angew, Physiol Enschl Arbeitsphysiol* 1961; 19:35–55.

Rozier CK, Elder JD, Brown M: Prevention of atrophy by isometric exercise of a casted leg. *J Sports Med* 1979; 19:191–194.

Strafford DE, Petrofsky JS: Interactions between fatiguing and nonfatiguing isometric contractions. *J Appl Physiol* 1981; 51:399–404.

Svendsen DA, Matyas TA: Facilitation of the isometric maximum voluntary contraction with traction. *Am J Phys Med* 1983; 62:27–36.

Temkin LP: Isometric exercise: A danger or a benefit? *Ariz Med* 1986; 6:380–383.

Isotonic Exercise

Alexander JF, Martin SL, Metz K: Effects of a four-week training program on certain physical components of conditioning male university students. *Res Q* 1968; 39:16–23.

American College of Sports Medicine: The recommended quantity and quality of exercise for developing and maintaining fitness in healthy adults. *Med Sci Sports* 1978; 10:7–10.

Arendt EA: Strength development: A comparison of resistive exercise techniques. *Contemp Orthop* 1984; 9:67–72.

Aronen JG, Regan K: Decreasing the incidence of recurrence of first time anterior shoulder dislocations with rehabilitation. *Am J Sports Med* 1984; 12:283–291.

Barney VS, Bangerter BL: Comparison of three programs of progressive resistance exercises. *Res Q* 1961; 32:138–146.

Berger RA: Effect of varied weight training programs on strength. *Res Q* 1962; 33:168–181.

Berger RA: Comparison of static and dynamic strength increases. *Res Q* 1962; 33:329–333.

Bonde-Petersen F, Hendriksson J, Knuttgen HG: Effect of training with eccentric muscle contractions on skeletal muscle metabolites. *Acta Physiol Scand* 1973: 88:564–570.

Brady TA, Cahill BR, Bodnar LM: Weight training-related injuries in the high school athlete. *Am J Sports Med* 1982; 10:1–5.

Brinkhorst RA, Hof MA: Overload and training: Compensatory hypertrophy and contraction characteristics of *M. plantaris* in female and male rats. *Experientia* 1973; 29:671–673.

Brown C, Wilmore JH: The effect of maximal resistance training on the strength, and body composition of women athletes. *Med Sci Sports* 1973; 5:29–33.

Capen EK: The effect of systematic weight training on power, strength, and endurance. *Res Q* 1950; 21:83–93.

Capen EK, Bright JA, Line PA: The effects of weight training on strength, power, endurance, and anthropometric measurements on a select group of college females. *J Assoc Phys Mental Rehabil* 1961; 15:169–173.

DeLorme TL, Watkins AL: Techniques of progressive resistance exercise. *Arch Phys Med* 1948; 29:263–273.

DeLorme TL: Restoration of muscle power by heavy resistance exercises. *J Bone Joint Surg* 1945; 27:645–667.

Dickinson A, Bennett KM: Therapeutic exercise. *Clin Sports Med* 1985; 4:417–429.

Edelstein ES: Changes in strength, girth, and adipose tissue of the upper arm resulting from daily and alternate day progressive weight training, thesis, Temple University, 1964.

Fleck SJ, Schutt RC Jr: Types of strength training. *Clin Sports Med* 1985; 4:159–168.

Foran B: Advantages and disadvantages of isokinetics, variable resistance and free weights. *NSCA J* 1985; 7:24–25.

Gettman LR, Cutler LA, Strathman TA: Physiologic changes after 20 weeks of isotonic vs isokinetic circuit training. *J Sports Med* 1980; 20: 265–274.

Gettman LR, Pollock ML: Circuit weight training: A critical review of its physiological benefits. *Phys Sports Med* 1960; 9:44–60.

Hempel LS, Wells CL: Cardiorespiratory cost of the Nautilus Express Circuit. *Phys Sports Med* 1985; 13:82–97.

Katch FI, Drumm SS: Effects of different modes of strength training on body composition and anthropometry. *Clin Sports Med* 1986; 5:413–459.

Katch FI, Freedson PS, Jones CA: Evaluation of acute cardiorespiratory responses to hydraulic resistance exercise. *Med Sci Sports Exerc* 1985; 17:168–173.

Knight KL: Guidelines for rehabilitation of sports injuries. *Clin Sports Med* 1985; 4:405–416.

Knowlton GC, Bennett RL: Overwork. *Arch Phys Med* 1957; 38:18–20.

Kraemer W: Exercise prescription: Isotonic loading. *Nat Strength Conditioning Assoc J* 1984; 6:47.

Kusinitz I, Keeney CE: Effects of progressive weight training on health and physical fitness of adolescent boys. *Res Q* 1958; 29:294–301.

Leach RE, Stryker WS, Zohn DA: A comparative study of isometric and isotonic quadriceps exercise programs. *J Bone Joint Surg* 1965; 47A:1421–1426.

Mayhew JL, Gross PM: Body composition changes in young women with high resistance weight training. *Res Q* 1974; 45:433–440.

Nosse LJ, Hunter GR: Free weights: A review supporting their use in training and rehabilitation. *Athletic Training* 1985: 20:206–209.

O'Shea P: Effects of selected weight training programs on the development of strength and muscle hypertrophy. *Res Q* 1966; 37:95–102.

Oyster N: Effect of a heavy-resistance weight training program on college women athletes. *J Sports Med* 1979; 19:79–83.

Paulos L, Noyes FR, Grood E, et al: Knee rehabilitation after anterior cruciate ligament reconstruction and repair. *Am J Sports Med* 1981; 9:140–149.

Pencek R: Effects of weight training on body weight, body density and body fat, Master's thesis, Pennsylvania State University, 1966.

Pipes TV: Strength training modes: What's the difference? *Scholastic Coach* 1977; 46:96–124.

Pipes TV: Variable resistance versus constant resistance strength training in adult males. *Eur J Appl Physiol* 1978; 39:27–35.

Pipes TV, Wilmore JH: Isokinetic vs isotonic strength training in adult men. *Med Sci Sports* 1975; 7:262–274.

Rasch PJ, Morehouse LE: Effect of static and dynamic exercise on muscular strength and hypertrophy. *J Appl Physiol* 1957; 11:29–35.

Rasch PJ, Pierson WR: Some relationships of isometric strength, isotonic strength and anthropometric measures. *Ergonomics* 1963; 6:211–215.

Smith MJ, Melton P: Isokinetic versus isotonic variable-resistance training. *Am J Sports Med* 1981; 9:275–279.

Smith MJ: Muscle fiber type: Their relationship to athletic training and rehabilitation. *Clin Sports Med* 1985; 4:179–187.

Tanner JM: The effect of weight training on physique. *Am J Phys Anthropol* 1952; 10:427–460.

Telle JR, Gorman IJ: Combining weights with hydraulics. *NSCA J* 1985; 7:66–68.

Viewpoint: A response to Nautilus. *NSCA J* 1980; 2:42–43.

Viewpoint: Nautilus. *NSCA J* 1978; 1:17–19.

Williams M, Stutzman L: Strength variation throughout the range of joint motion. *Physiologie* 1969; 27:96–100.

Wilmore JH: Alterations in strength, body composition and anthropometric measurements consequent to 10-week weight training program. *Med Sci Sports* 1981; 6:133–138.

Wolf M: The Nautilus controversy. *NSCA J* 1981; 3:38–41.

Wolf MD: Viewpoint: A response to the Yessis critique of Nautilus: II. Policy statement. *NSCA J* 1980; 2:39.

Yessis M: A response to the reaction of Dr. Wolf to the Yessis critique of Nautilus. *NSCA J* 1981; 3:36–39.

Isokinetic Exercise

Abdenour TE: Patellofemoral rehabilitation. *Phys Sports Med* 1983; 11:207.

Addison R, Schultz A: Trunk strengths in patients seeking hospitalization for chronic low-back disorders. *Spine* 1980; 5:539–544.

Adeyanju K, Crews TR, Meadors WJ: Effects of two speeds of isokinetic training on muscular strength, power and endurance. *J Sports Med* 1983; 23:352–356.

Alderink GJ, Kuck DJ: Isokinetic shoulder strength of high school and college-aged pitchers. *J Orthop Sports Phys Ther* 1986; 7:163–172.

Alexander J, Molnar G: Muscular strength in children: Preliminary report on objective standards. *Arch Phys Med Rehabil* 1973; 54:424–427.

Alston W, Carlson KE, Feldman DG, et al: A quantitative study of muscle fatigue in the chronic low-back syndrome. *J Am Geriatr Soc* 1966; 14:1041–1047.

Appen L, Duncan PW: Strength relationship of knee musculature: Effects of gravity and sports. *J Orthop Sports Phys Ther* 1986; 7:232–235.

Armstrong LE, Winant DM, Swashey PR, et al: Using isokinetic dynamometry to test ambulatory patients with multiple sclerosis. *Phys Ther* 1983; 63:1274–1279.

Aronen JG, Regan K: Decreasing the incidence of recurrence of first time anterior shoulder dislocations with rehabilitation. *Am J Sports Med* 1984; 12:283–291.

Arvidsson E, Eriksson E, Haggmark T: Isokinetic

thigh muscle strength after ligament reconstruction in the knee joint: Results from a 5-10 year follow-up after reconstructions of the anterior cruciate ligament in the knee joint. *Int J Sports Med* 1981; 2:7–11.

Berg K, Glank D, Miller M: Muscular fitness profile of female college basketball players. *J Orthop Sports Phys Ther* 1985; 7:59–63.

Berkson N, Schultz A, Nachemson A, et al: Voluntary strengths of male adults with acute low back syndromes. *Clin Orthop* 1977; 129:84–95.

Bohannon RW, Larkin PA: Cybex II isokinetic dynamometer for the documentation of spasticity: Suggestions from the field. *Phys Ther* 1985; 65:46–47.

Bohannon RW, Lieber C: Cybex II isokinetic dynamometer for passive load application and measurement: Suggestion from the field. *Phys Ther* 1986; 66:1407.

Burnie J, Brodie DA: Isokinetics in the assessment of rehabilitation: A case report. *Clin Biomech* 1986; 1:140–145.

Caiozzo VJ, Perrine JJ, Edgerton VR: Training induced alterations of the in vivo force-velocity relationship of human muscle. *J Appl Physiol* 1981; 51:750–754.

Caldwell LS, Chaffin DB, Dukes-Dobos FN, et al: A proposed standard procedure for static muscle strength testing. *Am Ind Hyg Assoc J* 1974; 35:201–206.

Campbell DE, Glenn W: Foot-pounds of torque of the normal knee and the rehabilitated post-meniscectomy knee. *Phys Ther* 1979; 59:418–421.

Campbell DE, Glenn W: Rehabilitation of knee flexor and knee extensor muscle strength in patients with meniscectomies, ligamentous repairs, and chondromalacia. *Phys Ther* 1982; 62:10–15.

Chaffin DB: Ergonomics guide for assessment of human static strength. *Am Ind Hyg Assoc J* 1975; 36:505–511.

Chaffin DB: Human strength capability and low-back pain. *J Occup Med* 1974; 16:248–254.

Chaffin DB, Herrin GD, Keyserling WM: Pre-employment strength test. *J Occup Med* 1978; 20:403–408.

Clarkson PM, John J, Dextradeur D, et al: The relationships among isokinetic endurance, initial strength level, and fiber type. *Res Q Exerc Sport* 1982; 53:15–19.

Costain R, Williams AK: Isokinetic quadriceps and hamstring torque levels of adolescent female soccer players. *J Orthop Sports Phys Ther* 1984; 5:196–199.

Costill DL, Coyle EF, Fink WF, et al: Adaptations in skeletal muscle following strength training. *J Appl Phys* 1979; 43:96–99.

Coyle EF, Costill DL, Lesmes GR: Leg extension power and muscle fiber composition *Med Sci Sports* 1978; 10:12–15.

Coyle EF, Fiering DC, Rotkis TC, et al: Specificity of power improvements through slow and fast isokinetic training. *J Appl Physiol* 1985; 5:1437–1442.

Davies GJ: *A Compendium of Isokinetics in Clinical Usage and Rehabilitation Techniques,* ed 2. La Cross, S&S Publishers, 1984, pp 3–17, 80, 81.

Davies GJ, Gould JA: Trunk testing using a prototype Cybex II isokinetic dynamometer stabilization system. *J Orthop Sports Phys Ther* 1982: 3:164–170.

Davies GJ, Gould JA, Ross DE: Trunk extensor weakness in back problem patients: Objectively quantified using a prototype Cybex II trunk dynamometer testing system, in Davies GJ: *A Compendium of Isokinetics in Clinical Usage,* ed 2. LaCross, S&S Publishers, 1984, pp 321–325.

DeLateur BJ, Giaconi RM: Effect on maximal strength of submaximal exercise in Duchenne muscular dystrophy. *Am J Phys Med* 1979; 58:26–36.

Dibrezzo R, Gench BE, Hinson MM, et al: Peak torque values of the knee extensor and flexor muscles of females. *J Orthop Sports Phys Ther* 1985; 7:65–68.

Distefano V, Nixon JE, O'Neil R, et al: Pes anserinus transfer: An in vivo biomechanical analysis. *Am J Sports Med* 1977; 5:204–208. (Note: Reprint is available from Cybex.)

Dobyns JH, Sim FH, Linscheid RL: Sports stress syndromes of the hand and wrist. *AM J Sports Med* 1978; 6:236–254.

Dummer GM, Vacaro P, Clarke D: Muscular strength and flexibility of two female master swimmers in the eighth decade of life. *J Orthop Sports Phys Ther* 1985; 6:235–237.

English WR Jr, Young DR, Moss RE, et al: Chronic muscle over use syndrome in baseball. *Phys Sports Med* 1984; 12:111–115.

Eriksson E: Rehabilitation of muscle function after sport injury: Major problem in sports medicine. *Int J Sports Med* 1981; 2:1–6.

Esterson PS, Simons DA: Rehabilitation following patellofemoral surgery. *Orthop Rev* 1985; 14:59–73.

Falkel J: Plantar flexor strength testing using the Cybex isokinetic dynamometer. *Phys Ther* 1978; 58:847–850.

Fleming RE Jr, Blatz DJ, McCarroll JR: Lateral reconstruction for anterolateral rotatory instability of the knee. *Am J Sports Med* 1983; 11:303–307.

Garnica RA: Muscular power in young women after slow and fast isokinetic training. *J Orthop Sports Phys Ther* 1986; 8:1–9.

Gehlsen GM, Grigsby SA, Winant DM: Effects of an aquatic fitness program on the muscular strength and endurance of patients with multiple sclerosis. *Phys Ther* 1984; 64:653–657.

Gerald ES, Caiozzo VJ, Rubin BJ, et al: Skeletal muscle profiles among elite long, middle, and short distance swimmers. *Am J Sports Med* 1982; 14:77–82.

Gettman LR, Culter L, Strathman TA: Physiologic changes after 20 weeks of isotonic vs isokinetic circuit training. *J Sports Med* 1980; 20:265–274.

Gilliam TB, Sady SP, Freedson PS, et al: Isokinetic torque levels for high school football players. *Arch Phys Med Rehabil* 1979; 60:110–114.

Gleim GW, Micholas JA, Webb JN: Isokinetic evaluation following leg injuries. *Phys Sports Med* 1978; 6:75–82.

Glove TP, Sayers JM III, Kent BE, et al: Non-operative treatment of the torn anterior cruciate ligament. *J Bone Joint Surg* 1983; 65A:184–192.

Gore DR, Murray MP, Sepic SB, et al: Correlations between objective measures of function and a clinical knee rating scale following total knee replacement. *Orthopedics* 1986; 9:1363–1367.

Gould JA, Davies GJ: *Orthopaedic and Sports Physical Therapy.* St Louis, CV Mosby Co, 1985, p 193.

Gracovetsky S, Farfan H, Helleur C: The abdominal mechanism. *Spine* 1985; 10:317–323.

Gransberg L, Knutsson E: Determination of dynamic muscle strength in man with acceleration controlled isokinetic movements. *J Sports Med Phys Fitness* 1983; 23:352–356.

Greer M, Dimick S, Burns S: Heart rate and blood response to several methods of strength training. *Phys Ther* 1984; 64:179–183.

Grimby G: Progressive resistance exercise for injury rehabilitation: Special emphasis on isokinetic training. *Sports Med* 1985; 2:309–315.

Grimby G, Gustafsson E, Peterson L, et al: Quadriceps function and training after knee ligament surgery. *Med Sci Sports Exerc* 1980; 12:70–75.

Hamberg P, Gillquist J, Lysholm J, et al: The effect of diagnostic and operative arthroscopy and open meniscectomy on muscle strength in the thigh. *Am J Sports Med* 1983; 11:289–292.

Hansson TH, Bigos SJ, Wortley MK, et al: The load on the lumbar spine during isometric strength testing. *Spine* 1984; 9:720–724.

Harber P, SooHoo K: Static ergonomic strength testing in evaluation occupational back pain. *J Occup Med* 1984; 26:877–884.

Hasue M, Fujiwara M, Kikuchi S: A quantitative measurement of abdominal and back muscle strength. *Spine* 1980; 5:143–148.

Hill JA, Moynes DR, Yocum LA, et al: Gait and functional analysis of patients following patellectomy. *Orthopedics* 1983; 6:724–728.

Hoke B, Howel D, Stack M: The relationship between isokinetic testing and dynamic patellofemoral compression. *J Orthop Sports Phys Ther* 1983; 4:150–153.

Holmes JR, Alderink GJ: Isokinetic strength characteristics of the quadriceps femoris and hamstring muscles in high school students. *Phys Ther* 1984; 64:914–918.

Housh TJ, Thorland WG, Tharp GD, et al: Isokinetic leg flexion and extension strength of elite adolescent female track and field athletes. *Res Q Exerc Sports* 1984; 55:347–350.

Hunt GC, Fromherz WA, Danoff J, et al: Female transverse torque: An assessment method. *J Orthop Sports Phys Ther* 1986; 7:319–324.

Imwold CHJ, Rider RA, Haymes EM, et al: Isokinetic torque differences between college female varsity basketball and track athletes. *J Sports Med* 1983; 23:67–73.

Indelicato PA: Nonoperative treatment of complete tears of the medial collateral ligament of the knee. *J Bone Joint Surg* 1983; 65A:323–329.

Ivy JL, Withers RT, Maxwell BD, et al: Isokinetic contractile properties of the quadriceps with relation to fiber type. *Eur J Appl Physiol* 1981; 47:247–255.

Jenkins WL, Thackaberry M, Killian C: Speed-specific isokinetic training. *J Orthop Sports Phys Ther* 1984; 5:181–183.

Jensen JE, Conn RR, Hazelrigg G, et al: The use of transcutaneous neural stimulation and isokinetic testing in arthroscopic knee surgery. *Am J Sports Med* 1985; 13:27–33.

Johnson JH: A comparison of isokinetic and isotonic training for college women. *Am Corr Ther J* 1980; 34:176–181.

Johnson J, Siegel D: Reliability of an isokinetic movement of the knee extensors. *Res Q* 1978; 49:88–90.

Kanehisa H, Miyashita M: Effect of isokinetic muscle training on static strength and dynamic power. *Eur J Appl Physiol* 1983; 50:365–371.

Kelly JM, Gorney BA, Kalm KK: The effects of a collegiate wrestling season on body composition, cardiovascular fitness and muscular strength and endurance. *Med Sci Sports* 1978; 10:119–124.

Keyserling WM, Herrin GD, Chaffin DB: Isometric strength testing as a means of controlling medical incidents on strenuous jobs. *J Occup Med* 1980; 22:332–336.

Kirkendall DT, Bergfeld JA, Calabrese L, et al: Isokinetic characteristics of ballet dancers and the response to a season of ballet training. *J Orthop Sports Phys Ther* 1984: 5:207–211.

Knapik JJ, Mawdsley RH, Ramos MV: Angular specificity and test mode specificity of isometric and isokinetic strength training. *J Orthop Sports Phys Ther* 1983; 5:58–65.

Knutsson E, Martensson A: Action of dantrolene sodium in spasticity in low dependence on fusimotor drive. *J Neurol Sci* 1976; 29:195–212.

Krotkiewski M, Aniansson A, Grimby G, et al: The effect of unilateral isokinetic strength training on local adipose and muscle tissue morphology, thickness, and enzymes. *Eur J Appl Physiol* 1979; 42:271–281.

Laird CE Jr, Rozier CK: Toward understanding the terminology of exercise mechanics. *Phys Ther* 1979; 59:287–292.

Lander JE, Bates BT, Sawhill JA, et al: A comparison between free-weight and isokinetic bench pressing. *Med Sci Sports Exerc* 1984; 17:344–353.

Langrana NA, Lee KC, Mayott CW: Quantitative assessment of back strength using isokinetic testing. *Spine* 1984; 9:287–290.

Lankenner PA Jr, Micheli LJ, Clancy R, et al: Arthroscopic percutaneous lateral patellar retinacular release. *Am J Sports Med* 1986; 14:267–269.

Lankhorst GJ, Van de Stadt RJ, Van der Korst JK: The relationships of functional capacity, pain, and isometric and isokinetic torque in osteoarthrosis of the knee. *Scand J Rehabil Med* 1985; 17:167–172.

Larsson L, Grimby G, Karlsson J: Muscle strength

and speed of movement in relation to age and muscle morphology. *J Appl Physiol* 1979; 43:451–456.

Lennington KB, Yanchuleff TT: The use of isokinetics in the treatment of chondromalacia patellae: A case report. *J Orthop Sports Phys Ther* 1983; 4:176–178.

Lesmes GT, Costill DL, Coyle EF, et al: Muscles strength and power changes during maximal isokinetic training. *Med Sci Sports* 1978; 10:266–269.

Lipscomb AB, Johnston RK, Snyder RB, et al: Evaluation of hamstring strength following use of semitendinosus and gracilis tendons to reconstruct the anterior cruciate ligament. *Am J Sports Med* 1982; 10:340–342.

Little KD, Sinning WE: Reliability of maximal isokinetic strength and work measures. *Med Sci Sports Exerc* 1985; 17:247.

Lysholm J, Nordin M, Elstrand J, et al: The effect of a patella brace on performance in a knee extension strength test in patients with patellar pain. *Am J Sports Med* 1984; 12:110–111.

Malek MM: Arthroscopic lateral retinacular release: Functional results in series of 67 knees. *Orthop Rev* 1985; 14:55–60.

Manzione M, Pizzutillol PD, Peoples AB, et al: Meniscectomy in children: A long-term follow-up study. *Am J Sports Med* 1983; 11:111–115.

Marras WS, King AI: Measurement of leads on the lumbar spine under isometric and isokinetic conditions. *Spine* 1984; 9:176–187.

Mayer TG: Using physical measurement to assess low-back pain. *J Musculoskel Med* 1985; 2:44–59.

Mayer TG, Gatchell RJ, Kishno N, et al: Objective assessment of spine function following industrial injury: A prospective study with comparison group and one-year follow-up. *Spine* 1985; 10:482–493.

Mawsley RA, Knapik JJ: Comparison of isokinetic measurements with test repetitions. *Phys Ther* 1982; 62:169–172.

McNeill T, Warwick D, Andersson G, et al: Trunk strengths in attempted flexion, extension and lateral bending in healthy subjects and patients with low-back disorders. *Spine* 1980; 5:529–538.

Merrifield HH, Cowan RFG: Groin strain injuries in ice hockey. *J Sports Med* 1973; 1:41–42. (Note: Reprint may be obtained from Cybex.)

Miller LS, Donahur JR, Good RP, et al: The Magnuson-Stack procedure for treatment of recurrent glenohumeral dislocation. *Am J Sports Med* 1984; 12:133–137.

Mira AL, Markley K, Greer RB III: A critical analysis of quadriceps function after femoral shaft fracture in adults. *J Bone Joint Surg* 1980; 62A:61–67.

Moffroid MT, Whipple RH: Specificity of speed of exercise. *Phys Ther* 1970; 50:1692–1700.

Moffroid M, Whipple RH, Hofkosh J, et al: A study of isokinetic exercise. *J Am Phys Ther Assoc* 1969; 49:735–747.

Molnar GE, Alexander J: Objective quantitative muscle testing in children: A pilot study. *Arch Phys Med Rehabil* 1973; 54:224–228.

Molnar GE, Alexander J: Development of quantitative standards for muscle strength in children. *Arch Phys Med Rehabil* 1974; 55:490–493.

Moore M: Scouting the elite unbreakable football player. *Phys Sports Med* 1981; 9:131–135.

Morns A, Jussier L, Bell G, et al: Hamstring/quadriceps strength rations in collegiate middle-distance and distance runners. *Phys Sports Med* 1983; 11:71–77.

Moroz JS, Sale DG: Evaluation of the torque transducer of the Cybex II dynamometer. *Med Sci Sports Exerc* 1985; 17:247.

Morris JM, Benner G, Lucas DB: An electromyographic study of intrinsic muscles of the back in man. *J Anat* 1962; 96:509–516.

Morris MC, Brewster CE: Hamstring weakness after surgery for anterior cruciate injury. *J Orthop Sports Phys Ther* 1986; 7:310–313.

Mostardi RA, Porterfield JA, Greenberg B, et al: Musculoskeletal and cardiopulmonary characteristics of the professional ballet dancer. *Phys Sports Med* 1983; 11:53–61.

Mostardi RA, Porterfield JA, King S, et al: Pre-employment screening and cardiovascular intervention program. *J Orthop Sports Phys Ther* 1986; 8:42–45.

Murray MP, Jacobs PA, Mollinger LA, et al: Functional performance after excision of the vastus lateralis and vastus intermedius. *J Bone Joint Surg* 1983; 65A:856–859.

Nachemson AL, Lindh M: Measurement of abdominal and back muscle strength with and without low-back pain. *Scand J Rehabil Med* 1969; 1:60–63.

Nicholas JA, Strizak AM, Veras G: A study of thigh muscle weakness in different pathological states of the lower extremity. *Am J Sports Med* 1976; 4:241–248.

Nistor L: Surgical and non-surgical treatment of Achilles tendon rupture. *J Bone Joint Surg* 1981; 63A:394–399.

Noyes FR, Matthews DS, Mooar PA, et al: The symptomatic anterior cruciate deficient knee: II. The results of rehabilitation activity modification and counseling on functional disability. *J Bone Joint Surg* 1983; 65A:163–174.

Oberg B, Ekstrand J, Moller M, et al: Muscle strength and flexibility in different positions of soccer players. *Int J Sports Med* 1984; 5:213–216.

Olerund S, Wallenstein R, Olsson E: Muscle strength after bilateral femoral osteotomy: A case report. *J Bone Joint Surg* 1984; 66A:792–793.

O'Neill R: Prevention of hamstring and groin strain. *Athletic Training* 1976; 11:27–31.

Osternig LR, Bates BT, James SL: Patterns of tibial rotary torque in knees of healthy subjects. *Med Sci Sports Exerc* 1980; 12:195–199.

Parker MG: Calculation of isokinetic rehabilitation velocities for knee extensor. *J Orthop Sports Phys Ther* 1982; 4:32–35.

Parker MG, Ruhling RO, Holt D, et al: Descriptive analysis of quadriceps and hamstrings muscle torque in high school football players. *J Orthop Sports Phys Ther* 1983; 5:2–6.

Pedegana LR, Elsner RC, Roberts D, et al: The relationship of upper extremity strength to throwing speed. *Am J Sports Med* 1982; 10:352–354.

Pedersen O, Petersen R, Schack Staffedlt E: Back pain and isometric back muscle strength of workers in a Danish factory. *Scand J Rehabil Med* 1975; 7:125–128.

Pfeiffer RD, Francis RS: Effects of strength training on muscle development in pre-pubescent, pubescent, and post-pubescent males. *Phys Sports Med* 1986; 14:1345–1352.

Pipes TV, Wilmore JH: Isokinetic vs isotonic strength training in adult men. *Med Sci Sports* 1975; 7:L262–274.

Poulmedis P: Isokinetic maximal torque power of Greek elite soccer players. *J Orthop Sports Phys Ther* 1985; 6:293–295.

Prietto CA, Caiozzo VJ, Prietto PP, et al: Closed versus open partial meniscectomy: Postoperative changes in the force-velocity relationship of muscle. *Am J Sports Med* 1983; 11:189–194.

Puhl J, Case S, Fleck S, et al: Physical and physiological characteristics of elite volleyball players. *Res Q Exerc Sport* 1982; 53:257–262.

Pytel LJ, Kamon E: Dynamic strength testing as a predictor for maximal lifting. *Ergonomics* 1981; 24:663–672.

Quigley TB, Scheller AD: Surgical repair of ruptured Achilles tendon. *Am J Sports Med* 1980; 8:244–250.

Rankin JM, Thompson CBN: Isokinetic evaluation of quadriceps and hamstrings function: Normative data concerning body weight and sports. *Athletic Training* 1983, pp 110–114.

Richards JG, Cooper J: Implementation of an on-line isokinetic analysis system. *J Orthop Sports Phys Ther* 1982; 4:32–35.

Rosentsweig J, Hinson E, Hinson M: Comparison of isometric, isotonic and isokinetic exercise by electromyography. *Arch Phys Med Rehabil* 1972; 53:32–34.

Ross DE, Gould JA, Davies GJ: Comparative testing data: Standing vs seated positioning Cybex trunk testing, in Davies GJ: *A Compendium of Isokinetics in Clinic Usage*, ed 2. LaCrosse, S&S Publishers, 1985, pp 327–343.

Roxin LE, Venge P, Friman G: Variations in serum myoglobin after a 2-min isokinetic exercise test and the effects of training. *Eur J Appl Physiol* 1984; 53:43–47.

Sandor SM, Hart JAL, Oakes BW: Case study: Rehabilitation of a surgically repaired medial collateral knee ligament using a limited motion cast and isokinetic exercise. *J Orthop Sports Phys Ther* 1986; 7:154–158.

Sepega A, Minkoff J, Nicholas J, et al: Sport-specific performance factor profiling fencing as a prototype. *Am J Sports Med* 1978; 6:232–235.

Sapega AA, Nicholas JA, Sokolow D, et al: The nature of torque "overshoot" in Cybex isokinetic dynamometry. *Med Sci Sports Exerc* 1982; 14:368–375.

Schlinkman B: Norms for high school football players derived from Cybex data reduction computer. *J Orthop Sports Phys Ther* 1984; 5:183–188.

Seaborne D, Taylor AW: The effects of isokinetic exercise on vastus lateralis fibre morphology and biochemistry. *J Sports Med* 1981; 21:365–370.

Seaborne D, Taylor AW: The effect of speed on isokinetic exercise on training transfer to isometric strength in the quadriceps muscle. *J Sports Med* 1984; 24:183–188.

Shields CL Jr, Beckwith VA, Kurland HL: Comparison of leg strength training equipment. *Phys Sports Med* 1985; 13:49–56.

Shields CL Jr, Kerlan RK, Jobe FW, et al: The Cybex II evaluation of surgically repaired Achilles tendon ruptures. *Am J Sports Med* 1978; 6:369–372.

Sherman WM, Pearson DR, Plyley MJ, et al: Isokinetic rehabilitation following surgery: A review of factors which are important for developing physiotherapeutic techniques following knee surgery. *Am J Sports Med* 1982; 10:155–161.

Sherman WM, Plyley MJ, Pearson DR, et al: Isokinetic rehabilitation after meniscectomy: A comparison of two methods of training. *Phys Sports Med* 1983; 11:121–133.

Simmons JW, Rath D, Merta R: Calculation of disability using the Cybex II system. *Orthopedics* 1982; 5:181–185.

Smidt G, Herring T, Amundsen L, et al: Assessment of abdominal and back extensor strength: A quantitative approach and results for chronic low-back patients. *Spine* 1983; 8:211–219.

Smith DJ, Quinney HA, Senger HA, et al: Isokinetic torque outputs of professional and elite amateur ice hockey players. *J Orthop Sports Phys Ther* 1981; 3:42–47.

Smith MJ, Melton P: Isokinetic versus isotonic variable resistance training. *Am J Sports Med* 1981; 9:275–279.

Smith SS, Mayer TG, Gatchel RJ, et al: Quantification of lumbar function: I. Isometric and multispeed isokinetic trunk strength measures in sagittal and axial planes in normal subjects. *Spine* 1985; 10:757–764.

Smith CF: Physical management of muscular low-back pain in the athlete. *Can Med Assoc J* 1977; 117:632–635.

Sobush DC, Fehring RJ: Physical fitness of physical therapy students. *Phys Ther* 1983; 63:1266–1273.

Sockolov R, Irwin B, Dressendorfer RH, et al: Exercise performance in 6 to 11 year old boys with muscular dystrophy. *Arch Phys Med Rehabil* 1977; 58:195–201.

Stafford MG, Grana WA: Hamstring/quadriceps ratios in college football players: A high velocity evaluation. *Am J Sports Med* 1984; 12:209–211.

Steadman JR: Rehabilitation of the injuries. *Am J Sports Med* 1979; 7:147–149.

Steele V: Rehabilitation of the injured athlete. *Physiotherapy* 1980; 66:251–255.

Stonecipher DR, Catlin PA: The effect of a forearm strap on wrist extensor stength. *J Orthop Sports Phys Ther* 1984; 6:184–189.

St Pierre RK, Andrews L, Allman F, et al: The Cybex II evaluation of lateral ankle ligamentous reconstructions. *Am J Sports Med* 1984; 12:52–56.

Stoddard G: The physical rehabilitation of selected shoulder injuries. *Athletic Training* 1978; 13:34–40.

Stray-Gunderson J, Snell PG, Smith SS, et al: The systemic myocardial oxygen demand associated with an isokinetic trunk testing protocol. *Med Sci Sports Exerc* 1985; 17:207.

Strickler EM, Greene WB: Isokinetic torque levels in hemophiliac knee musculature. *Arch Phys Med Rehabil* 1984; 65:766–770.

Suzuki N, Endo S: A quantitative study of trunk muscle strength and fatigability in the low-back pain syndrome. *Spine* 1983; 8:1–2.

Suzuki N, Selichi E: A quantitative study of trunk muscle strength and fatigability in the low-back pain syndrome. *Spine* 1983; 8:69–74.

Tegner Y, Lysholm J, Lysholm M, et al: A performance test to monitor rehabilitation and evaluate anterior cruciate ligament injuries. *Am J Sports Med* 1986; 14:156–159.

Teige RA, Indelicato PA, Kerlan RK, et al: Iliotibial band transfer for anterolateral rotatory instability of the knee. *Am J Sports Med* 1980; 8:223–227.

Thompson NN, Gould JA, Davies GJ, et al: Descriptive measures of isokinetic trunk testing. *J Orthop Sports Phys Ther* 1985; 7:43–49.

Thorblad J, Ekstrand J, Hamberg P, et al: Muscle rehabilitation after arthroscopic meniscectomy with or without tourniquet control: A preliminary randomized study. *Am J Sports Med* 1985; 13:133–135.

Thorstensson A, Arvedson A: Trunk muscle testing and low-back pain. *Scand J Rehabil Med* 1982; 14:69–75.

Thorstensson A: Muscle strength, fibre types and enzyme activities in man. *Acta Physiol Scand* 1976; 98(suppl 449):7–38.

Thorstensson A, Karlsson J: Fatigability and fibre composition of human skeletal muscle. *Acta Physiol Scand* 1976: 98:318–322.

Thorstensson A, Nilsson J: Trunk muscle strength during constant velocity movements. *Scand J Rehabil Med* 1982; 14:P61–75.

Timm KE, Patch DG: Case study: Use of the Cybex II velocity spectrum in the rehabilitation of post-surgical knees. *J Orthop Sports Phys Ther* 1985; 6:347–349.

Tippett SR: Lower extremity strength and active range of motion in college baseball pitchers: A comparison between stance leg and kick leg. *J Orthop Sports Phys Ther* 1986; 98:10–14.

Tippett SR: A case study: Lenox Hill bracing for post-operative total knee replacement. *J Orthop Sports Phys Ther* 1984; 5:265–268.

Troup JDG, Chapman AF: The strength of the flexor and extensor muscles of the trunk. *J Biomech* 1969; 2:49–62.

Vanswearinger JM: Measuring wrist muscle strength. *J Orthop Sports Phys Ther* 1983; 4:217–228.

Vitti GJ: The effects of variable training speeds on leg strength and power. *Athletic Training* 1984; 19:26–30.

Wagner MB, Vignos PJ Jr, Fonow DC: Serial isokinetic evaluations used for a patient with scapuloperoneal muscular dystrophy. *Phys Ther* 1986; 66:1110–1113.

Walmsley RP, Swann I: Biomechanics and physiology of muscle strengthening. *Physiotherapy (Canada)* 1976; 28:197–200.

Watkins MP, Harris BA, Wender S, et al: Effect of patellectomy on the function of thedriceps and hamstrings. *J Bone Joint Surg* 1983; 65A:390–395.

Watkins MP, Harris BA, Kozlowski BA: Isokinetic testing in patients with hemiparesis: A pilot study. *Phys Ther* 1984; 64:184–189.

Wiktorsson-Moller M, Oberg BV, Ekstrand J, et al:

Effects of warming up, massage, and stretching on range of motion and muscle strength in the lower extremity. *Am J Sports Med* 1983; 11:249–252.

Winter DA, Wells RP, Orr GW: Errors in the use of isokinetic dynamometers. *Eur J Appl Physiol* 1981; 46:397–408.

Wong DLK, Glasheen-Wray M, Andrews LF: Isokinetic evaluation of the ankle invertors and evertors. *J Orthop Sports Phys Ther* 1984: 5:246–252.

Wright KE: An Orthotron knee rehabilitation program. *Athletic Training* 1979; 14:232–233.

Wyatt MP, Edwards AM: Comparison of quadriceps and hamstring torque values during isokinetic exercises. *J Orthop Sports Phys Ther* 1981; 3:48–56.

OTHER MODALITIES

Continuous Passive Motion

Akeson WH, Woo SL-Y, Amiel D, et al: The connective tissue response to immobility: Biomechanical changes in periarticular connective tissue of the immobilized rabbit knee. *Clin Orthop* 1973; 93:356–362.

Arm SW, Pope MH, Johnson RJ, et al: The biomechanics of anterior cruciate ligament rehabilitation and reconstruction. *Am J Sports Med* 1984; 12:8–18.

Blokker CP, Rorabeck CH, Bourne RB: Tibial plateau fractures: An analysis of results in treatment in 60 patients. *Clin Orthop* 1984; 182:193–199.

Cabaud HE, Chatty A, Gildengorin V, et al: Exercise effects on the strength of the rat anterior cruciate ligament. *Am J Sports Med* 1979; 8:79–85.

Coutts RD, Toth C, Kaita JH: The role of continuous passive motion in the rehabilitation of the total knee patient, in Hungerford DS, Krackow KA, Kenna KA (eds): *Total Knee Arthroplasty: A Comprehensive Approach.* Baltimore, Williams & Wilkins Co, 1983, pp 126–132.

Eriksson E, Haggmark T: Comparison of isometric muscle training and elecrical stimulation supplementing isometric muscle training in recovery after major knee ligament surgery. *Am J Sports Med* 1979; 7:169–171.

Frank C, Akeson WH, Woo SL-Y, et al: Physiology and therapeutic value of passive joint motion. *Clin Orthop* 1984; 185:113–125.

Gelberman RH, Menon J, Gonsalves M, et al: The effects of mobilization on the vascularization of healing flexor tendons in dogs. *Clin Orthop* 1980; 153:283–289.

Gelberman RH, Van de Berg JS, Lundborg GN, et al: Flexor tendon healing and restoration of the gliding surface. *J Bone Joint Surg* 1983; 65A:70–80.

Godfrey CM, Jayawardena H, Quance TA, et al: Comparison of electro-stimulation and isometric exercise in strengthening the quadriceps muscle. *Physiotherapy (Canada)* 1979; 31:2–4.

Goodship AE, Lanyon LE, McFie H, et al: Functional adaptation of bone to increased stress. *J Bone Joint Surg* 1979; 61A:539–546.

Gould N, Donnermeyer D, Pope M, et al: Transcutaneous muscle stimulation as a method to retard disuse atrophy. *Clin Orthop* 1982; 164:215–220.

Greene WB: Use of continuous passive slow motion in the postoperative rehabilitation of difficult pediatric knee and elbow problems. *J Pediatr Orthop* 1983; 3:419–423.

Hall MC: Cartilage changes after experimental immobilization of the knee joint of the young rat. *J Bone Joint Surg* 1963; 45A:36–44.

Hohl M: Tibial condylar fractures. *J Bone Joint Surg* 1967; 49A:1455–1467.

Inoue M, Gomez M, Hollis V, et al: Medial collateral ligament healing repair vs nonrepair. *Trans Orthop Res Soc* 1986; 11:78.

Laros GS, Tipton CM, Cooper RR: Influence of physical activity on ligament insertions in the knee of dogs. *J Bone Joint Surg* 1971; 53A:275–286.

Morrissey MC, Brewster CE, Shields CL, et al: The effects of electrical stimulation on the quadriceps during postoperative knee immobilization. *Am J Sports Med* 1985; 13:40–45.

Noyes FR: Functional properties of knee ligaments and alterations induced by immobilization. *Clin Orthop* 1977; 123:210–242.

Noyes FR, Butler DL, Paulos LE, et al: Intra-articular cruciate reconstruction: I. Perspectives on graft strength vascularization and immediate motion after replacement. *Clin Orthop* 1983; 172:71–77.

Noyes FR, Torvik PJ, Hyde WB, et al: Biomechanics of ligament failure. *J Bone Joint Surg* 1974; 56A:1406–1418.

O'Driscoll SW, Kumar A, Salter RB: The effect of continuous passive motion on the clearance of a hemarthrosis from a synovial joint. *Clin Orthop* 1983; 176:305–311.

O'Driscoll SW, Salter RB: The induction of neochondrogenesis in free intra-articular periosteal autografts under the influence of continuous passive motion. *J Bone Joint Surg* 1984: 66A:1248–1257.

Perry CR, Evans LG, Rice S, et al: A new surgical approach to fractures of the lateral tibial plateau. *J Bone Joint Surg* 1984; 66A:1236–1240.

Porter B: Crush fractures of the lateral tibial tubercle: Factors influencing the prognosis. *J Bone Joint Surg* 1970; 52B:676–687.

Salter RB, Bell RS, Keeley FW: The protective effect of continuous passive motion on living articular cartilage in acute septic arthritis. *Clin Orthop* 1981; 159:223–247.

Salter RB, Ogilvie-Harris DJ: Healing of intra-articular fractures with continuous passive motion. AAOS Instruction Course Lectures. 1979, pp 102–117.

Salter RB, Simmonds DF, Malcolm BW, et al: The biological effect of continuous passive motion on the healing of full-thickness defects in articular cartilage. *J Bone Joint Surg* 1980; 62A:1232–1251.

Woo SL-Y, Ritter MA, Amiel D, et al: The biomechanical and biochemical properties of swine tendon: Long-term effects of exercise on the digital extensors. *Connect Tissue Res* 1980; 7:177–183.

Stationary Bicycle

Arms SW, Pope MH, Johnson RJ, et al: The biomechanics of anterior cruciate ligament rehabilitation and reconstruction. *Am J Sports Med* 1984; 12:8–18.

Cabaud HE, Chatty A, Gildengorin V, et al: Exercise effects on the strength of the rat anterior cruciate ligament. *Am J Sports Med* 1980; 8:79–86.

Costill DL, Fink WJ, Habansky AJ: Muscle rehabilitation after knee surgery. *Phys Sports Med* 1977; 5:71–75.

Ericson MO, Bratt A, Nisell R, et al: Load moments about the hip and knee joints during ergometer cycling. *Scand J Rehabil Med* 1986; 18:165–172.

Ericson MO, Ekholm J, Svensson O, et al: The forces on ankle joint structures during ergometer cycling. *Foot Ankle* 1985; 6:135–142.

Ericson MO, Nisell R: Tibiofemoral joint forces during ergometer cycling. *Am J Sports Med* 1986; 14:285–290.

Ericson MO, Nisell R, Ekholm J: Varus and valgus loads on the knee joint during ergometer cycling. *Scand J Sports Sci* 1984; 6:39–45.

Eriksson E: Sports injuries of the knee ligaments: Their diagnosis, treatment, rehabilitation, and prevention. *Med Sci Sports* 1976; 3:133–144.

Goldfuss AJ, Moorehouse CA, LeVeau BF: Affect of muscular tension on knee stability. *Med Sci Sports* 1973; 4:267–271.

Henning CE, Lynch MA, Glick KR: An in vivo strain gage study of elongation of the anterior cruciate ligament. *Am J Sports Med* 1985; 13:22–26.

McLeod WD, Blackburn TA: Biomechanics of knee rehabilitation with cycling. *Am J Sports Med* 1980; 8:175–182.

Paulos L, Noyes FR, Grood E, et al: Knee rehabilitation after anterior cruciate ligament reconstruction and repair. *Am J Sports Med* 1981; 9:140–149.

Steadman JR: Nonoperative measures for patellofemoral problems. *Am J Sports Med* 1979; 7:374–375.

Index

GRIMSBY COLLEGE

LIBRARY

NUNS CORNER, GRIMSBY